nMRCGP
Practice Cases:
Clinical Skills Assessment

Raj Thakkar
BSc (Hons) MBBS MRCGP MRCP (UK)
General Practitioner
Buckinghamshire

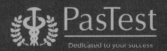

PasTest
Dedicated to your success

© 2009 PASTEST LTD
Egerton Court
Parkgate Estate
Knutsford
Cheshire
WA16 8DX

Telephone: 01565 752000

First Published 2009

ISBN: 1905635524

           9781905635528

A catalogue record for this book is available from the British Library.

The information contained within this book was obtained by the author from reliable sources. However, while every effort has been made to ensure its accuracy, no responsibility for loss, damage or injury occasioned to any person acting or refraining from action as a result of information contained herein can be accepted by the publishers or author.

PasTest Revision Books and Intensive Courses

PasTest has been established in the field of postgraduate medical education since 1972, providing revision books and intensive study courses for doctors preparing for their professional examinations.

Books and courses are available for the following specialties:
MRCGP, MRCP Parts 1 and 2, MRCPCH Parts 1 and 2, MRCPsych, MRCS, MRCOG Parts 1 and 2, DRCOG, DCH, FRCA, PLAB Parts 1 and 2.

For further details contact:

PasTest, Freepost, Knutsford, Cheshire WA16 7BR

Tel: 01565 752000 Fax: 01565 650264

www.pastest.co.uk enquiries@pastest.co.uk

Text prepared by Carnegie Book Production, Lancaster

Printed and bound in the UK by Page Bros., Norwich

CONTENTS

ABOUT THE AUTHOR

Raj Thakkar BSc (Hons) MBBS MRCGP MRCP (UK), gained his neuroscience and medical degrees from University College London. During his vocational training in the Oxford deanery, he won the national GP enterprise award, registrar division. He currently works as a GP partner in Buckinghamshire, where his special interest is cardiovascular medicine, and as a hospital practitioner in echocardiography. Raj is a freelance writer and GP advisor for several medical magazines.

ABOUT THE CONTRIBUTORS

Peter Havelock MBBS, FRCGP graduated from St Mary's London in 1970 and became a general practitioner in Wooburn Green, Buckinghamshire. He has been involved in teaching for many years, being a trainer, course organiser, RCGP examiner and Associate Director in the Oxford Deanery. His special interests within teaching have been teaching and learning around the Doctor/Patient Consultation. He has been the author of many papers and books about the subject and has run courses for hundreds of trainers and registrars around the UK.

Alice Barnes BSc, BMBS, DCH, DRCOG, nMRCGP graduated from Nottingham Medical School in 2004. Having just completed General Practice training in Buckinghamshire she is currently a Senior Registrar with the Oxford Deanery where she is developing a specialist interest in Family Planning. Her particular area of interest is in teenage sexual and reproductive health.

INTRODUCTION

Today's GPs are faced with the challenge of a rapidly evolving NHS. As well as having to keep up with these radical changes, doctors are required to practise safe and effective medicine taking into account best practice, evidence-based medicine, and clinical governance while considering the financial pressures the NHS is under.

General practice has seen dramatic changes in recent times. The new General Medical Services (GMS) contract, Choose and Book, practice-based commissioning and the polyclinic debate have transformed medicine in the community into a dynamic, unique, and fast-moving profession.

Irrespective of these changes, general practitioners (GPs) must remain patient-focused, think holistically, and consult using specialised techniques tailored to the individual. Effective consulting remains at the hub of general practice, and is the focus of the clinical skills assessment (CSA) component of the nMRCGP®. A number of unique skills and attributes are required to consult effectively, and these are tested in the CSA.

To select those most suited to meet the challenges of modern general practice, candidates are required to pass a robust set of key stages. Once successful, trainee GPs rotate through hospital specialties before entering into the final stage of training at a training practice. During that time trainees will learn a number of skills including, the art of consulting, performing focused clinical examinations, the management of risk and uncertainty, and the management of both acute and chronic diseases. In addition they will gain experience in business and practice management. By the end of GP training it is hoped that registrars will be able to learn and practise independently. Many of these essential skills are assessed through the, now compulsory, nMRCGP assessment.

The nMRCGP replaces both the old summative assessment and the MRCGP® examination. As it is an 'exit' examination, success is essential to gain the Certificate of Completion of Training (CCT) in general practice, entry onto the General Medical Council (GMC) GP register, and of course college membership.

The nMRCGP assessment, which is based on the GP curriculum, consists of three components; firstly the workplace-based assessment (WPBA: ongoing appraisal throughout general practice training, information collated using portfolio), secondly the applied knowledge test (AKT: computer based examination. Various question styles are used including: single best answers, extended matching, data interpretation and questions based on pictures. The knowledge tested includes: clinical medicine, organisational aspects of general practice, legal issues, major clinical trials and evidence based practice), and finally the CSA (live examination). This book concerns itself with the CSA component of the nMRCGP.

The CSA is far more than a test of consulting skills, although candidates are required to consult using models such as Pendleton et al, Neighbour, and Silverman. As it is a live simulated surgery, it also examines a candidate's ability to assess and manage medical and social problems. Assessment may involve appropriate clinical examination while management requires application of accepted guidelines and current evidence.

The first two chapters of this book have been written by Peter Havelock; a highly experienced GP, an ex-college examiner, and co-author of numerous and highly acclaimed texts on consultation skills including The Consultation[1] and The New Consultation[2] (Pendleton et al). He describes the examination itself followed by an invaluable account of the consultation skills required to be successful in the CSA. Dr Alice Barnes, recently successful in completing the nMRCGP, then gives a unique personal insight into the CSA and how to succeed. Finally, two practice examinations offer an opportunity to role play, teasing out various skills required to pass the assessment. The cases presented in this book are designed to reflect real-life general practice. Each practice case has basic information taken from the patient's case notes, similar to those you are likely to encounter in the CSA. A blank page has been included to brainstorm any thoughts based on the notes. Attached to each case is a brief for the role player. The text printed in bold italic is information that the role player should only volunteer if specifically asked about. A marking sheet with teaching points and clinical notes are discussed after each case.

To make the most of the book, the cases should be practised under examination conditions. You may want to practise a whole examination all at once or, alternatively, discuss each case after you have role played, teasing out the various issues and then role playing again using different consultation styles and techniques until you have found one that works for you. The book may be used in small group teaching with fellow registrars. Your revision, however, shouldn't stop with this book; every case you see in your daily practice should be considered a CSA case, after all, the nMRCGP is designed not test your knowledge of esoteric medicine, but to reflect everyday, high-quality general practice.

REFERENCES

(1) Pendleton D, Schofield T, Tate P and Havelock P (1984) *The Consultation: An Approach to Teaching and Learning.* Oxford: Oxford University Press.

(2) Pendleton D, Schofield T, Tate P and Havelock P (2003). *The New Consultation.* Oxford: Oxford University Press.

ABBREVIATIONS

ACE	angiotensin-converting enzyme
ACE-1	ace inhibitor
ACR	albumin : creatinine ratio
A&E	accident and emergency department
AF	atrial fibrillation
AKT	applied knowledge test
AV	atrio-ventricular node
AVRT	atrio-ventricular re-entry tachycardia
BMI	body mass index
BNF	British National Formulary
BP	blood pressure
BTS	British Thoracic Society
CbD	case based discussion
CCF	congestive cardiac failure
CCT	certificate of completion of training
CEO	chief executive officer
CFC	chlorofluorocarbons
CLL	chronic lymphoblastic leukaemia
COPD	chronic obstructive pulmonary disease
COT	consultant observation tool
CRP	C-reactive protein
CSA	clinical skills assessment
CVD	cardiovascular disease
CXR	chest X-ray
DEXA	dual-energy X-ray absorptiometry
DVT	deep vein thrombosis
ECG	electrocardiogram
EER	experimental event rate
eGFR	estimated glomerular filtration rate
ESR	erythrocyte sedimentation rate
FBC	full blood count

FEV$_1$	forced expiratory volume in 1 second
FP10	blank prescription
FVC	forced vital capacity
GFI	glomerular filtration rate
GI	glycaemic index
GMC	General Medical Council
GMS	General Medical Services
HAP	hospital anxiety and depression score
Hb	haemoglobin
HCA	health care assistant
hCG	human chorionic gonadotropin
HDL	high density lipoprotein
HRT	hormone replacement therapy
IB204	obligations for doctor to issue certificate
ICD	internal cardioverter-defibrillator
ICS	inhaled corticosteroids
JVP	jugular venous pressure
LABA	long lasting β antagonists
LVF	left ventricular failure
MA	meta-analysis
MAOI	monoamine oxidase inhibitor
MCH	mean corpuscular haemoglobin
MCV	mean corpuscular volume
MED 3	blank certificate
MED 5	sickness certificate
MI	myocardial infarction
MMR	measles, mumps and rubella
MRC	Medical Research Council
MRI	magnetic resonance imaging
MRSA	methicillin-resistant *Staphylococcus aureus*
MSF	multi-source feedback
MSU	midstream urine
NICE	National Institute for Health and Clinical Excellence
NNT	number needed to treat

nocte	every night
NTA	National Treatment Agency
NSAID	non-steroidal anti-inflammatory drug
NSTEMI	non-ST-elevation myocardial infarction
OA	osteoarthritis
OCD	obsessive–compulsive disorder
od	*omni die* (once daily)
PCL	posterior cruciate ligament
PCT	primary care trust
PCOS	polycystic ovary syndrome
PCR	polymerase chain reaction
PE	pulmonary embolus
PEFR	peak expiratory flow rate
PID	pelvic inflammatory disease
PMB	post menopausal bleeding
PMETB	Postgraduate Medical Education and Training Board
PMR	polymyalgia rheumatica
POP	progestogen-only pill
PR	per rectal
prn	as required
PSA	prostate-specific antigen
PT	prothrombin time
PUVA	psoralens + UVA
QALY	quality-adjusted life-year
qds	*quarter die sumendum* (to be taken four times a day)
QOF	Quality and Outcomes Framework
RCGP	Royal College of General Practitioners
RCT	randomised controlled trial
RICE	rest, ice, compression and elevation
RRR	relative risk reduction
RSV	respiratory syncytial virus
SCC	squamous-cell carcinoma
SD	standard deviation
SIGN	Scottish Intercollegiate Guidelines Network

SLE	systemic lupus erythematosus
SLS	selected list scheme
βhCG	beta-human chorionic gonadotrophin
SMART	Sameterol Muticentre Asthma Research Trial
SOB	shortness of breath
SSRI	selective serotonin reuptake inhibitor
STEMI	ST-elevation myocardial infarction
STI	sexually transmitted infection
T3	triiodothyronine
T4	thyroxine
TB	tuberculosis
tds	*ter die sumendum* (to be taken three times a day)
TED	thromboembolic deterrent
TENS	transcutaneous electrical stimulation
TFT	thyroid function test
TIA	transient ischaemic attack
TSH	thyroid-stimulating hormone
2WW	two weeks wait
U&Es	urea and electrolytes
UTI	urinary tract infection
URTI	upper respiratory tract infection
UVA	long-wavelength ultraviolet (light)
VEGF	vascular endothelial growth factor
WCC	white cell count
WPBA	workplace-based assessment
WPW	Wolff-Parkinson-White Syndrome
WOMAC	Western Ontario and McMaster Universities Index of Osteoarthritis

Chapter 1
The CSA examination: history and overview

Peter Havelock

> **Box 1: Definition of the purpose of the CSA**
>
> "An assessment of the doctor's ability to integrate and apply appropriate clinical, professional, communication and practical skills in general practice."
>
> www.rcgp-curriculum.org.uk/nmrcgp/csa.aspx

The CSA examination is a clinical consulting skills examination, based on cases from general practice, with the role players as patients and experienced MRCGP assessors. The assessment is able to provide a pre-determined, standardised level of challenge to the candidates. It is derived from the video component and the simulated surgery of the previous MRCGP. The advantage of the CSA as an assessment process is that it assesses the clinical skills of the candidates in a wide range of situations. The CSA triangulates information from the other aspects of the MRCGP; the workplace-based assessment, and the applied knowledge test. The use of simulated patients is a well tried technique, and is valid for testing clinical skills. It is essential that the case production is quality assured and the role players and the assessors are well trained and monitored. The CSA is based on the Royal College of General Practitioners' (RCGP's) curriculum, and the cases are selected to include the wide spectrum found in everyday general practice. The RCGP website describes the CSA and points out those areas of the curriculum that are particularly tested.

The CSA tests mainly from the following areas of the curriculum:

Primary care management – recognition and management of common medical conditions in primary care.

Problem-solving skills – gathering and using data for clinical judgment, choice of examination, investigations and their interpretation. Demonstration of a structured and flexible approach to decision making.

Comprehensive approach – demonstration of proficiency in the management of co-morbidity and risk.

Person-centred care – communication with patient and the use of recognised consultation techniques to promote a shared approach to managing problems.

Attitudinal aspects – practising ethically with respect for equality and diversity, with accepted professional codes of conduct.

The CSA will also test:

Clinical practical skills– demonstrating proficiency in performing physical examinationinations and using diagnostic/therapeutic instruments.

The role players are professionally trained and will play the same role about 28 times in a day. Their roles are written to enable them to respond to the appropriate questions and communication skills from the candidate. They need to be treated with respect and courtesy and the examination needs to be done carefully and with empathy; they have no assessment role. The assessors are unobtrusive and their only task is to mark the candidates.

THE MECHANISMS OF THE CSA

The candidates will all be tested at the same purpose modified test centre in Croydon. The CSA is run a number of times a year (see www.rcgp.org. uk), and candidates may apply any time within the ST3 year and take it more than once. The format is: 13 simulated patients (12 are assessed and another is a pilot case: you won't know which one is the pilot); each patient is accompanied by an assessor who will remain with the same case each time. There is an initial briefing and you will be shown to your room. In the room will be the case notes for each patient in order, blank prescriptions (FP10), and blank certificates (Med 3). The role players and assessors will be shown to your room; the cases last 10 minutes with a 2 minute break between cases. A buzzer will sound to mark the start and the end of the cases; there will be a 15 minute break after the seventh case with an opportunity to go to the toilet and have refreshments. A clinical examination may be required, but the patient may decline to be examined; there are no intimate examinations. Which clinical examination you choose, and how you perform will be marked. There might be important physical signs.

You can write on the notes provided, but they have no part in the marking and are not to be removed from the room. The prescriptions or certificates are to be given to the role player, and they may be marked.

THE MARKING SCHEDULE

Each case is marked in three domains:

1. data-gathering, technical and assessment skills
2. clinical management skills
3. interpersonal skills.

DATA-GATHERING, TECHNICAL AND ASSESSMENT SKILLS

Gathering and using data for clinical judgement, choice of examination, investigations and their interpretation. Demonstrating proficiency in performing physical examinations, and using diagnostic and therapeutic instruments.

CLINICAL MANAGEMENT SKILLS

The recognition and management of common medical conditions in primary care. Demonstrating a structured and flexible approach to decision making. Demonstrating the ability to deal with multiple complaints and co-morbidity. Demonstrating the ability to promote a positive approach to health.

INTERPERSONAL SKILLS

Demonstrating the use of recognised communication techniques to understand the patient's illness experience and develop a shared approach to managing problems. Practising ethically with respect for equality and diversity, in line with the accepted codes of professional conduct.

All three domains have equal weighting and the assessor uses word pictures to help them decide which grade to give for each domain; then uses this information to make a judgment on the case overall. On the marking schedule there is a box for serious concerns which, fortunately, is used only rarely. The assessor will also make notes for feedback to the candidates.

CHAPTER 1

Chapter 2
Consultation skills in the CSA

Peter Havelock

INTRODUCTION

The clinical skills assessment (CSA), as the name indicates, is focused on the work the GPs do in their consulting rooms with patients. This was very well described nearly 50 years ago by Sir James Spence; and it is the candidate's competency at this that the CSA strives to assess.

Box 1

"The essential unit of medical practice is the occasion when, in the intimacy of the consulting room or sick room, a person who is ill or believes himself to be ill, seeks the advice of a doctor whom he trusts. This is a consultation and all else in the practice of medicine derives from it. The purpose of the consultation is that the doctor, having gathered his evidence, shall give explanation and advice."

Spence J[1]

As Box 1 suggests, the consultation is the cornerstone of general practice. The average GP registrar will have more than 4000 consultations in 12 months, and if they continue a career in general practice will conduct more than 100 000 face to face consultations. It is not surprising that the nMRCGP has a very strong focus on the consultation and therefore in the teaching; over the ST3 year the consultation is constantly discussed and assessed. The CSA should not be looked at in isolation because many of the areas of the curriculum covered in the CSA are also covered in the workplace-based assessment. Clearly the consultant observation tool (COT) is focused on the consultation; the feedback in these sessions is essential in developing the registrar's skills in the consultation. It is thus important to do many more COT assessments than the minimal. The COT assessment criteria give the registrars clear guidance on the elements of 'an effective consultation'.

CHAPTER 2

Box 2: The COT assessment criteria

- Encourage the patient's contribution

- Respond to cues

- Place complaint in appropriate psychosocial contexts

- Explore patient's health understanding

- Include or exclude likely relevant significant condition

- Make an appropriate physical or mental state examination

- Make an appropriate working diagnosis

- Explain the problem in appropriate language

- Seek to confirm the patient understands

- Make an appropriate management plan

- Give the patient the opportunity to be involved in significant management decisions

- Make effective use of resources

- Specify conditions and interval for follow-up.

The sensible registrar will work at each of the criteria to understand the evidence for it, to master the strategies and skills that are needed to achieve it, and to practise their skills in their day-to-day consultations.

THE RELATIONSHIP OF THE CSA TO THE RCGP CURRICULUM

Over the last few years there has been a great deal of work within the RCGP to create and coordinate the GP curriculum with the end point assessment of GP training. This has been stimulated by the Postgraduate Medical Education and Training Board (PMETB) who have set standards for the training of doctors. Information and an explanation of the work of this important organisation can be found on their web site, www.pmetb.org.uk where the start of the page 'about us' is:

'PMETB is the independent regulatory body responsible for postgraduate medical education and training. We ensure that postgraduate training for doctors is of the highest standard.' Their remit covers all the Royal Colleges.

The GP Curriculum should be well known to all trainee doctors considering a career in general practice and is found on the RCGP website, www.rcgp-curriculum.org.uk. There are specific areas of the curriculum that are particularly assessed by the CSA and some of the domains more obviously covering the whole area of consultation skills and are:

- **Primary care management** – recognition and management of common medical conditions in primary care.

- **Problem-solving skills** – gathering and using data for clinical judgment, choice of examination, investigations and their interpretation, and the demonstration of a structured and flexible approach to decision making.

- **Comprehensive approach** – demonstration of proficiency in the management of co-morbidity and risk.

- **Person-centred care** – communication with patient and the use of recognised consultation techniques to promote a shared approach to managing problems.

- **Attitudinal aspects** – practising ethically with respect for equality and diversity, with accepted professional codes of conduct.

- **Clinical practical skills** – demonstrating proficiency in performing physical examination and using diagnostic/therapeutic instruments.

In this chapter I will not be going into the detail of these aspects of the curriculum, but it is essential that candidates are aware of them early in their training and have realised what knowledge and skills they need to learn and what attitudes are important in helping a consultation be effective. It is obvious that people learn best when they are clear what it is that they have to learn; GP trainees need to be clear about the GP curriculum and use it daily to drive their learning.

CHAPTER 2

HOW TO USE ALL YOUR ST3 YEAR TO DO WELL IN THE CSA CONSULTATION SKILLS

In the last paragraph I suggested that the GP registrar should be steeped in the RCGP curriculum, but I recognise that it can be seen as a mammoth task. Do not be put off but take it in bite-size pieces. The place to start is in the first two sections of the core and extended statements of the curriculum documents (www.rcgp-curriculum.org.uk) They are:

- Being a GP.

- The general practice consultation.

These will give the trainee a clear idea on what to learn. How to learn is a different matter and the Curriculum guide for Learners and Teachers from the RCGP is a very good start. It is recognised that different learners have different preferences on how they learn, but it is clear that they learn best when different learning methods or modalities are combined, eg by seeing, listening, talking and doing; and the same coherent messages are drawn from each.

Kolb (1984) described how people learn:

- Experience: learning by involvement.

- Reflective: learning by reviewing.

- Generalisation/theorist: learning by reading and discussion.

- Experiential or testing: learning through activities.

People can learn in many different ways, but by adulthood most people have demonstrated a preferred learning style. Nevertheless, learning involves several processes integrating activity with reflection, the discovery of new ideas and experimentation to see how our performance might be improved.

I will use the four points on the learning cycle as starting points for the learner; an entry point into the learning, not the place that they stay.

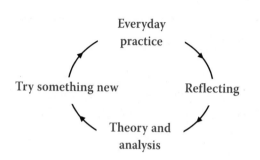

Fig. 1 Learning Cycle (after Kolb 1984)[2]

Everyday practice, for **the activist**, is the place to start. This is using the 20 plus face to face consultations each working day and, as they are going on, thinking about the patients – why is this patient bringing these symptoms to me today?

Peter Tate, who managed the MRCGP panel so well for many years, described this as developing a curiosity about the patient. The way to find out is not lots of questions, but really active listening. The skills are listed in figure 2, but the underlying skill is for the doctor to hear what the patient says and how they say it ; then work out with the patient why they are saying it.

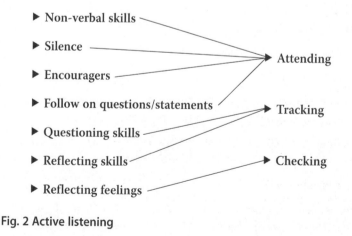

Fig. 2 Active listening

The **activist** can then use other aspects of the consultation to try new things and new ideas: but I am getting into the areas for the **experiential learner**.

The **reflective learner** might also start with the day-to-day consultation, but might wish to take the reflection further and use video feedback at an early stage. There are a number of published methods of doing this (Pendleton *et al* 2003[3]; Neighbour 1987[4]), but an easy place to start is using the COT criteria and getting help from the educational supervisor.

There is a lot of scope for the **generalist/theoretical learner** to start because the theoretical base of effective consulting is now vast and detailed. Probably, as suggested, the best starting place is the second chapter of the RCGP curriculum to get a simple overview; there is further reading indicated there. There are often articles in the current journals about different aspects of the consultation as it is of importance to all doctors regardless of their specialty. As well as reading discussion of cases with other clinicians, observing consultations can give an overview to the **generalist learner** .

The **experiential learner** will like to start with trying out new ideas in the consultation. These ideas might come from the trainer or from reading or discussion. There is a time and place to try out new skills: first thing Monday morning is probably not ideal. Introducing new skills needs planning:

• Start at a quiet time.

• Be clear what you are trying to do.

• Make small changes.

• Don't be put off by the patient's initial reaction (it is probably new for them too and might need some explanation).

• Continue to practise a skill until it stops feeling awkward for you; get the words right until you feel comfortable with them.

• Enjoy experimenting.

The reader will see from these starting points that there are artificial boundaries between the 'learning types'. It requires moving around the learning cycle many times and not staying in one area. Using all the opportunities within the training is essential to develop the skills to pass the CSA. Use the day release to get new approaches to the consultation and to get feedback from your peers; use the tutorials to cover areas that affect the consultation, eg when discussing diabetes ask your trainer how they manage the new diabetic when informing them of the diagnosis. I have already mentioned COTs and along with the case based discussion (CbD) they provide a rich source of feedback that can develop your consultations. Patient feedback and the results of your multi-source feedback (MSF) might give you pointers to develop your consultation skills. Your reading and discussions will give you skills and strategies that you might like to try in your consultations; make these into clear action plans and introduce them into your consultations.

Developing your consultation is like any skill that you might learn, eg learning the guitar or improving your wind-surfing. Firstly, it is getting clarity about what it is you are trying to learn; secondly, trying it out and getting feedback on your performance and thirdly practising, practising and practising. The practice stage is often lost, and the improvement is not maintained. It is important when you practise to get the changes that you wish to make unconscious, so you don't need to keep trying to remember questions; they just come naturally.

SPECIFIC PREPARATION FOR THE CSA CONSULTATION SKILLS

As the time draws near for your CSA what is there to be done in the way of 'revision' or 'swatting'? It is really important to remember that, unlike written examinations, this is a test of clinical skills where the candidate needs to turn to the consulting room as a solid base of preparation. Use each and every consultation as a potential examination station: imagine that you are being observed and shed any incorrect or sloppy habits; follow-up on clues presented, and hone your skills of reflection and analysis.

It is important at an early stage to encourage and welcome the more challenging consultations in your consulting room. Many doctors, particularly registrars, ignore clues that get them into difficult areas:

CHAPTER 2

Patient A	'... and I seem to be getting much more irritable recently.'
Doctor	' Uh uh. How is your sleeping?'
Patient B	'... and it is very distressing.'
Doctor	'I wouldn't worry. It will be fine.'
Patient C	'... and since then I have felt so tired.'
Doctor	'I will do some blood tests to make sure that you are ok.'

All three of these patients have given the doctor clues that he has chosen to ignore. The doctor will say that they will ask the questions next time, but the next consultation is another occasion and the discussion will be about sleep patterns or blood test results. The moment will be lost when the possible responses could have been:

To patient A	'Tell me about the irritable feelings.'
To patient B	'Why is it distressing?'
To patient C	'Talk to me about this tiredness' or 'How did the tiredness start?'

Ignored cues in the day-to-day consultation are often lost forever and in the CSA they will lose the candidate marks.

IN THE EXAMINATION

It is important to treat every patient as though they are in your consulting room; be respectful and friendly. Stand up when you first meet the patient, welcome them and ensure you address them by their name. Some patients may be blind, deaf or have other disabilities; they should be dealt with appropriately, guiding them or helping them to their seat if required. Do not 'show off' to the observer, that is a disaster. Interact with each patient appropriately even though the examination brief might be a clinical skill, eg examine the patient's knee and use those skills that you have been developing over your training:

- Really listen to the patient.

- Make the history focused.

- Make your explanations clear and jargon free, also succinct to save time – time is wasted by the doctor talking too much.

- Check out understanding and ask for any questions.

- Be aware of the patient's body language and react appropriately to it.

As well as being closely involved in the process of the consultation and using the above strategies and skills, it is important to have awareness of that process as it progresses:

- Be aware of the time.

- Try and get a flow throughout each consultation.

- Be logical and systematic.

Summarising the information you have collected and checking it out with the patients are helpful ways of gathering your thoughts.

REFERENCES

[1] Spence J (1960).The need for understanding the individual as part of the training and function of doctors and nurses. In *The Purpose and Practice of Medicine*. Oxford: Oxford University Press: 271–280.

[2] Kolb D (1984). *Experiential learning: Experience as a source of learning and development.* Englewood Cliffs: Prentice Hall.

[3] Pendleton D, Schofield T, Tate P and Havelock P (2003).*The New Consultation*. Oxford: Oxford University Press.

[4] Neighbour R (1987). *The Inner Consultation: how to develop effective and intuitive consulting skills.* Lancaster: Kluwer Academic Press.

Chapter 3
A personal experience

Alice Barnes

If you let it, the CSA can hover over your GP registrar year like a black cloud. It doesn't need to. The RCGP has spent time and energy perfecting this examination to make sure it does exactly what it says on the tin. It assesses you 'doing the day job', just as it should. So, if you structure your registrar year using all possible resources and prepare properly for both the AKT and CSA, there should be no surprises when it comes to the day of the assessment.

Here are some 'top tips' of how to succeed in the CSA.

BEFORE THE DAY

DON'T PREPARE FOR THE CSA IN ISOLATION

It is difficult to 'revise' for these examinations in the way you may have done for other more traditional written assessments. I would suggest that preparation for the CSA should be an ongoing project and an integral part of daily life as a GP trainee.

DON'T NEGLECT THE KNOWLEDGE ASPECT

The GP curriculum is huge and the range of possible topics vast – just like a normal surgery. You are not expected to know every tiny detail of every separate topic. But you do need to be able to convince the examiner that, whatever your knowledge or experience is in a particular subject area, you know how to approach clinical problems competently and safely.

Don't make the mistake of assuming the CSA is purely a test of your communication skills. It isn't. Your knowledge base is just as important. Focus your revision on topics you find difficult or those you're least experienced in. Here are some simple ways you can use your surgery time as preparation:

- After each surgery keep a logbook of cases or topics you found difficult and why.

- Read up on the clinical aspects **the same day** if at all possible.

- Discuss learning points with your trainer at your next de-brief session or tutorial to build on your knowledge base and consolidate learning.

It's all about active and learning throughout your training posts.

REMEMBER YOUR EXAMINATION SKILLS

It is a good time to go back to basics. Dust off your medical school textbooks and for each system spend time thinking about what you're doing and why. Practise your examinations on unsuspecting friends and family. Ask your trainer to watch you do them; discipline yourself to do proper examinations in your consultations as if it were the real thing. Be sensible though. You can't do every medical test under the sun in 10 minutes. GP examinations need to be targeted and focused. It might be useful to write down a pro forma for each system examination to help you to think things through logically.

FIND CONSULTATION MODELS THAT SUIT YOU, AND PRACTISE THEM

Early in the registrar year, learn about the different consultation models and think about what works best for you. It's OK to dip into a number of different models and piece together your preferred approach. Be strict with yourself, and set yourself challenges in each surgery (or at least each time you video) to work on a particular area of your consultation style. For instance, in one surgery you could focus on different ways of negotiating shared management plans with patients. Prior to the CSA, each surgery should be treated like an examination. If you do this, by the time the CSA comes around, your consultations will be well-structured and patient-centred.

USE YOUR TRAINER

Joint surgeries and use of COT, video assessments, and role playing are great ways for your trainer to see how you are doing, and for you to practise what you've learnt in front of an expert. Whilst this may feel daunting, you will really benefit from their input. Another benefit of joint surgeries is that you get used to having a third person in the consultation, as there will be in the CSA. It puts you on the spot in a different way and makes you put some of the techniques you've read about into practice.

PUT UP CRIB SHEETS IN YOUR CONSULTING ROOM

Tacked to the wall, out of the sight of my patients, I had little crib sheets detailing the structure of my 'perfect' consultation. Obviously you can't follow them exactly, but they are useful as a prompt if you're floundering. For instance, for the ideas, concerns, and expectations areas I had my favourite phrases highlighted so I could glance up at them quickly. Questions such as – 'Have you had any thoughts as to what's causing your symptoms?' This gets you into the habit of using the phrases within your consultations on a day-to-day basis. In this way, patient-centred consulting styles will become second nature by the time you sit the CSA. It is a good idea to get used to seeing patients in 10 minutes well before the CSA.

USE THE BOOKS AND CHALLENGE YOURSELF WITH ROLE PLAY

Case-based revision books for the CSA are a great resource if you use them properly. Don't just read them cover to cover but work with a colleague or your trainer to actually act some of the cases out. Role playing as a 'patient' for your colleagues helps to get you thinking again about how you would approach a given station. Many of the books, like this one, include guidelines and knowledge required to manage the case successfully. This is invaluable in the few weeks leading up to your CSA.

CHAPTER 3

MAKE SURE YOU KNOW THE DEADLINES

Make sure you know when the examinations are and when you can register for them. Be aware that the deadlines can vary depending on which sessions you apply for.

USE THE RCGP WEBSITE

Keep up to date. You'll find useful information on the RCGP website about the structure of the examination, some example cases, and what equipment you need to bring with you. Make sure you've got all your equipment ready well in advance of the day of the examination. Be sure you're using it properly – another reason why joint surgeries or videos are a good idea.

ORGANISE YOUR TRAVEL PLANS FOR THE EXAMINATION

It may not sound important, but make sure you can get to the assessment centre without any traumas on the day of the examination. If that means staying in a hotel the night before, so be it. There are plenty of places to stay nearby that are reasonably priced.

ON THE DAY

Stay calm. By now you've done all the hard work and the CSA should be a formality!

TRY TO RELAX

I used to hate it when people told me to relax, but it does work. The centre is comfortable, the staff are friendly, and there to help. Water, tea, and coffee are provided. Once you arrive, you will go into a room with all the other candidates for a briefing – nothing daunting, it just takes you through the structure of the examination and timings. Remember you are not allowed to take anything into the examination; even watches or stop-watches. All your equipment has to be in a clear plastic bag (provided) and everything else goes in your locker which you'll be taken to after the briefing.

GET USED TO YOUR ROOM

After the briefing you will be shown to your 'consulting room' and given a few minutes to settle in. On the desk you'll find pencils and all manner of forms (blood/X-ray forms, peak expiratory flow charts (PEFR), prescription pads, and medical certificates): a clock is in easy view. Then there are the case notes. My advice would be to read only one case at a time. If you flick through you're likely to panic and get overwhelmed. Read the small print and highlight anything you think is particularly important. There may be useful clues there.

THE ACTORS ARE EXCELLENT

When you are used to your surroundings just get ready to do a 'normal' surgery. An odd sounding buzzer will ring, and the first patient will knock on the door and be followed in by the examiner. Ignore the examiner who will try and sit out of your line of view as much as possible. Be nice to the patients/actors, just as you normally would be. Be polite and courteous, introduce yourself and then get going.

TIME IS SHORT

But no shorter than a normal surgery, so just do your best. If a patient comes in with deep, difficult issues, go with it. Don't try and rush things to tick all the boxes. Just make the best possible use of time. On the other hand, don't draw things out unnecessarily. If the case seems straightforward and you finish early that's fine. Just run through your checklist structure, and then end the consultation. By finishing just a little early it gives you a longer break between patients – a much needed breather.

EXAMINATIONS

You may be required to examine any system on the day. If you feel an intimate examination would be appropriate, offer this to the examiner and patient in the CSA. Say something like, 'normally I would proceed to do a rectal examination'. Clearly they will stop you, but at least they know you are thinking about it. Don't be thrown if you are offered a manikin to examine however. Think about how you'd approach that kind of situation in a CSA station.

USE YOUR TIME BETWEEN PATIENTS

These precious 2 minutes are vital for keeping you sane on the day. Take stock: have a breather. Then put all that has happened behind you, and read the next set of case notes. Stamina is an important component of this examination. In one of my breaks I made the mistake of feeling sorry for myself with my head in my hands. It meant I didn't read the next set of case notes properly and missed out on an important hint for a hidden clue, which I may have got otherwise.

THANK GOODNESS FOR THE COFFEE BREAK

Halfway through the examination, you will be ushered out of your room for a coffee and loo break. (You will find that even trips to the toilet have to be accompanied by an invigilator.) Spend time giving your brain a rest, and try to take your mind off the cases you've done so far. Talk about the weather or the news headlines, anything but the cases! Use the time to re-charge your batteries, forget what's gone before and concentrate on what's coming.

REMEMBER ALTERNATIVE CONSULTATIONS

Be prepared for being rushed out of your room to do a telephone consultation. If this happens, stay in role and don't get flummoxed – even if it seems a bit artificial. During your preparations think about how you'd handle the following consultations in the CSA:

- telephone consultations.

- consultations with a member of staff about a patient or colleague problem.

- consultations with family members about patients (a great way to test your understanding of confidentiality and/or consent).

- consulting a deaf/blind person.

- consulting a patient with learning difficulties with their carer.

- paediatric consultations (either with parents or young adolescents).

- There is a broad range, and any of them could be included. Take heart from the fact that as a GP you'll have coped with these problems before.

ABOVE ALL, BE YOURSELF

Try to treat the CSA as if it were normal surgery and make sure you have plans to celebrate when it's all over. You will deserve a pat on the back.

Lots and lots of luck!

Chapter 4
Example case

INTRODUCTION

Each case in this book has been designed to bring out particular skills and behaviours required for the CSA and hence independent practise. The format and style of the cases seen in this book reflect those one could expect in the CSA.

In the exam, you will be given a brief set of notes for each case you will encounter during your simulated surgery. Prior to the patient entering your room, a few minutes are allowed to study the notes and you are well advised to make brief notes (which are not marked) on what questions you may want to ask, your examination, management strategies and interpersonal skills you want to demonstrate. A page has been included with each case in this book for you to brainstorm any thoughts you have. Keep an eye on your watch; you have no more than 10 minutes per patient.

You could ask a colleague or friend to role play the patient and ideally another GP or fellow registrar to observe your effort. Videoing your consultation will provide you with unique insight into your own consulting behaviours.

A set of notes for the patient have also been included with each case. You, as the doctor, should not look at the patient notes until after you have completed the case. The patient notes have information which is readily volunteered to you (in black) and information that is only expressed if you specifically ask for it is printed in bold italic.

Welcome the patient and introduce yourself, asking how you can help them. The patient notes instruct the role player on what their opening statement should be. You should then consult in a patient-centred way, examining appropriately (respecting the patient at all times) and managing using evidence-based practice and accepted guidelines.

Once the case is complete, it is important to reflect on how well you did and how you may improve your performance. Ask the patient role player and the observer for their feedback. Review your videos, if you recorded the consultation, and appraise your own effort. What are your learning points? Role-play different consultation techniques over and over until you are satisfied you have mastered them. Have you consulted in a patient-centred way? Are your examination skills slick, if not, practice until they are. Do you know how to manage the cases, do you need to revise guidelines and management strategies?

Tips

✓ Behave as you would during a 'normal' surgery. Welcome the patient appropriately, introduce yourself, be courteous and unless otherwise instructed, offer how you may help the patient today.

✓ Follow well known consultation models such as *The New Consultation* (**Pendleton** *et al*) [1] or *The Inner Consultation* (**Roger Neighbour**)[2].

CHAPTER 4

INSTRUCTIONS TO CANDIDATE (CASE NOTES)

You have recently joined the practice as a salaried GP and have never met this patient before.

Name	Sharon Walker
Age	27
Past medical history	Nil
Current medication	Nil
Social History	Single
	Smoker

The last entry in the notes by practice nurse:

Palpitations. Intermittent. No chest pain.

Currently well.

Plan – bloods, ECG and refer to GP.

The electrocardiogram (ECG) is shown in figure 3. All of the blood tests were normal.

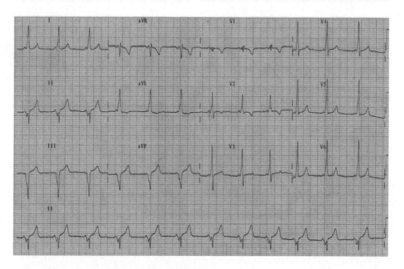

Fig. 3 Abnormal ECG – WPW syndrome

BRAINSTORM

Palpitations, ask about character, how long they last, regular or irregular, triggering factors

Does she get chest pain/dizziness/SOB?

Examine heart

Thyroid state?

What are patients ideas/concerns/expectations?

Does patient know about WPW?

Refer cardiology, is patient ok with this?

Follow up

Tips

- ✓ It is important not to fudge your way through the consultation if you don't understand what the results mean; have you been in a similar situation in your everyday practice? How have you managed it? It is far safer and more appropriate to admit to the patient you need to take some advice from a colleague, who may be another GP or a hospital doctor, than to make the wrong decision.

- ✓ Keep your cool! You have 10 minutes for each consultation. As in real life, there are no 'time outs'.

- ✓ Practise the cases in this book under examination conditions. Don't cheat by looking at the role player briefs until you have finished the case!

Role player information printed in bold italic should not be offered by the patient unless specifically asked for.

CHAPTER 4

INSTRUCTIONS TO ROLE PLAYER (PATIENT)

NOT TO BE SEEN BY THE CANDIDATE

Opening statement:

'Hello Doctor, I have come to the get the results of my heart tracing and blood tests.'

Patient background:

You are Sharon Walker, a 27-year-old dental nurse, who is anxious to get her test results. You had a heart tracing (ECG) and some blood tests after seeing the nurse for palpitations which you have been experiencing intermittently for the last 6 months.

The palpitations make you feel dizzy and breathless but never cause chest pain.

They start and stop suddenly, feel very fast and may last for up to 20 minutes at a time.

You drink a lot of caffeine and smoke 20 cigarettes per day.

You have been smoking for the last 5 years.

You would like help in giving up smoking

You don't feel depressed and enjoy life in general.

You don't drink alcohol or take illicit drugs.

Your weight is stable, and your bowels and periods are normal.

You are otherwise well, have no ongoing medical problems and don't take any regular medications.

You are allergic to penicillin: this causes a rash.

You are worried that you may collapse and die like your father did.

Your father died after suffering a heart attack 8 months ago. He was a heavy smoker.

You live with your mother and younger brother and enjoy swimming and badminton.

NOTES

DATA-GATHERING, TECHNICAL AND ASSESSMENT SKILLS

- In general, in a patient with a history of palpitations it is imperative to ascertain the nature of her symptoms. How long has she had them for? How frequently do they occur? How long do they last? Are there any trigger factors, eg caffeine, illicit drugs?

- Does she have any symptoms or signs of thyroid disease? Is there a family history of sudden cardiac death, or any other cardiac or thyroid disease? Does she experience chest discomfort, dizziness (or collapse) or breathlessness (sinister signs)?

- It is important to explain to the patient that you need to examine her heart, and check she is happy for you to do so. Check her pulse rate and ensure she is in sinus rhythm (feel pulse for at least 15 seconds).Measure her blood pressure and auscultate the praecordium to assess for structural cardiac disease. The standard way to take blood pressure is shown in figure 4 and figure 5 (see also British Hypertension Society www.bhsoc.org/how_to_measure_blood_pressure.stm)

- However, it would be impossible in a 10 minute consultation for you to spend 5 minutes (as recommended) taking her blood pressure. Examiners should accept a valid blood pressure, as long as she is relaxed and her arm is at heart level. If her blood pressure is raised it would be reasonable to take a second reading. If consistently high it should be re-checked at another consultation, perhaps with the practice nurse. If agreeable her heart should be examined without her clothes, but keeping under-garments on. You must ask permission for this. If she declines, which is likely for the purposes of the CSA, auscultate through her clothes.

CHAPTER 4

BLOOD PRESSURE MEASUREMENT
WITH ELECTRONIC BLOOD PRESSURE MONITORS

- The patient should be seated for at least 5 minutes, relaxed and not moving or speaking
- The arm must be supported at the level of the heart. Ensure no tight clothing constricts the arm
- Place the cuff on neatly with the indicator mark on the cuff over the brachial artery. The bladder should encircle at least 80% of the arm (but not more than 100%)
- Most monitors allow manual blood pressure setting selection where you choose the appropriate setting. Other monitors will automatically inflate and re-inflate to the next setting if required
- Repeat three times and record measurement as displayed. Initially test blood pressure in both arms and use arm with highest reading for subsequent measurement

CUFF SIZES

Indication	Width (cm)*=	Length (cm)*=	BHS Guidelines Bladder width & length (cms)*	Arm circ. (cm)*
Small Adult/Child	10 – 12	18 – 24	12 x 18	<23
Standard Adult	12 – 13	23 – 35	12 x 26	<33
Large Adult	12 – 16	35 – 40	12 x 40	<50
Adult Thigh Cuff **	20	42		<53

*The range for columns 2 and 3 are derived from recommendations from the British Hypertension Society (BHS), European Hypertension Society (ESH) and the American Heart Association. Columns 4 and 5 are derived from only the BHS guidelines.
** Large bladders for arm circumferences over 42cm may be required
= Bladders of varing sizes are available so a range is provided for each indication (applies to columns 2 and 3)

POINTS TO NOTE:

If checking against a mercury sphygmomanometer the blood pressure may differ slightly between devices.

It is good practice to occasionally check the monitor against a mercury sphygmomanometer or another validated device.

It is important to have a monitor calibrated according to manufacturer's instruction.

Fig. 4 Blood pressure measurement with electronic blood pressure monitors

Fig. 5 Blood pressure measurement with mercury blood pressure monitors

Reproduced with kind permission of the British Hypertension Society

CHAPTER 4

BLOOD PRESSURE MEASUREMENT WITH MERCURY BLOOD PRESSURE MONITORS

- The patient should be seated for at least 5 minutes, relaxed and not moving or speaking
- The arm must be supported at the level of the heart. Ensure no tight clothing constricts the arm
- Place the cuff on neatly with the centre of the bladder over the brachial artery. The bladder should encircle at least 80% of the arm (but not more than 100%)
- The column of mercury must be vertical, and at the observers eye level
- Estimate the systolic beforehand:
  a. Palpate the brachial artery
  b. Inflate cuff until pulsation disappears
  c. Deflate cuff
  d. Estimate systolic pressure
- Then inflate to 30mmHg above the estimated systolic level needed to occlude the pulse
- Place the stethoscope diaphragm over the brachial artery and deflate at a rate of 2-3mm/sec until you hear regular tapping sounds
- Measure systolic (first sound) and diastolic (disappearance) to nearest 2mmHg

CUFF SIZES

Indication	Width (cm)*=	Length (cm)*=	BHS Guidelines	Arm circ. (cm)*
			Bladder width & length (cms)*	
Small Adult/Child	10 – 12	18 – 24	12 x 18	<23
Standard Adult	12 – 13	23 – 35	12 x 26	<33
Large Adult	12 – 16	35 – 40	12 x 40	<50
Adult Thigh Cuff **	20	42		<53

*The range for columns 2 and 3 are derived from recommendations from the British Hypertension Society (BHS), European Hypertension Society (ESH) and the American Heart Association. Columns 4 and 5 are derived from only the BHS guidelines.

** Large bladders for arm circumferences over 42cm may be required

= Bladders of varing sizes are available so a range is provided for each indication (applies to columns 2 and 3)

POINTS TO NOTE:

The date of next servicing should be clearly marked on the sphygmomanometer (6 monthly).

All maintenance necessitating handling of mercury should be conducted by the manufacturer or specialised service units.

Anaeroid manometers tend to deteriorate and need regular checking. In many instances aneroid monitors cannot be corrected accurately therefore they should not be used as a substitute for mercury sphygmomanometers.

Tip

✓ Remember this is a CSA, not a medical school or MRCP examination! You are not required to perform a full cardiovascular examination.

- You don't necessarily have to examine her on a couch, although that would be ideal.

- In this case the diagnosis is evident from the ECG: **Wolff-Parkinson-White syndrome**(WPW). Of course, computer interpretations are not always correct!

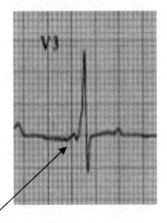

Fig. 6 Short PR interval and delta wave

- Irrespective of the diagnosis, it is still important to ask about chest pain, dizziness, and breathless. Much of the consultation should concentrate on explaining what WPW is and how she should be managed, particularly given her anxiety.

- Discussion about her job and lifestyle is important. Her job, as a dental nurse, may put her or her patients in physical danger if she were to collapse. A discussion about her concerns should be had in order to consider her health beliefs.

CLINICAL MANAGEMENT SKILLS

- You may want to discuss what you know about WPW, but a detailed knowledge would not be expected in the CSA

- WPW syndrome can occur in isolation or with structural heart disease, such as mitral valve prolapse and hypertrophic cardiomyopathy. It may cause serious and life threatening arrhythmias. Drugs such as digoxin are contra-indicated in this condition.

- The patient should be advised not to put herself in danger, eg riding a bike, climbing, swimming, particularly as she experiences dizziness or collapse.

- As far as the CSA is concerned, the most important medical management is to refer the patient to a cardiologist. It is likely she will have ambulatory ECG monitoring and as she is symptomatic ablation may be offered. It is prudent to explain what is going to happen next, so she knows what to expect. What are her expectations? Is she still happy for you to refer her to a cardiologist?

- It is important that she seeks advice if she gets sustained palpitations, chest pain, dizziness, breathlessness or is otherwise concerned (safety-net). Loss of consciousness is an ominous symptom and she may be admitted if this occurs.

- Discussion about her smoking is appropriate if she wishes. Explore what her views are on smoking, whether she is a pre-contemplator (in which case there should be a discussion about the dangers of smoking, perhaps anchoring the conversation around her father's smoking habits), or if she would like help to quit smoking. Of course, this may be a whole consultation in itself. In this case, a brief discussion and follow-up is all that you can offer.

- She should have appropriate follow-up to ensure her cardiac symptoms haven't deteriorated and/or to discuss the outcome of the cardiology assessment.

CHAPTER 4

INTERPERSONAL SKILLS

- She looks anxious; this is a non-verbal cue, and it may be worth commenting 'You look worried…'

- WPW is a difficult condition to explain to a patient; it is important to explain the condition in way she understands, to check understanding, and to give her opportunities to ask questions. You may want to describe WPW using drawings.

- If you are not sure about it be honest and explain it's an uncommon condition that requires a cardiology opinion. You may offer to send her some information in the post or to give her a website link, eg www.patient.co.uk. Write down 'Wolff-Parkinson-White' if she thinks she may forget it and wants to look it up on trusted websites.

- What are her ideas, concerns and expectations?

- She may think she has the same condition as her father. What does she think may happen to her?

- Asking whether she agrees with a specialist referral is still appropriate. Not referring would be unsafe, but she still needs to agree.

- Does she have worries about what the cardiologists may say and do?

NOTES ON WOLFF-PARKINSON-WHITE SYNDROME[3]

The three most common accessory pathways associated with paroxysmal tachycardias are the bundle of Kent, the Mahaim pathway and the James pathway. In these conditions, extra electrical conduits exist between the atrial and ventricular myocardium allowing pre-excitation of the ventricular muscle and, in some cases, a short PR interval and delta wave on the ECG. Re-entry tachycardias may result from anterograde electrical activity along the atrio-ventricular (AV) node and retrograde conduction through the accessory pathways resulting in a circus rhythm.

In the Wolff-Parkinson-White (WPW) syndrome, the accessory pathway is entirely separate from the AV node whereas Mahaim fibres arise within the AV node or the bundle of His and terminate in the ventricular myocardium. Only part of the AV node is bypassed by Mahaim fibres and hence the PR interval tends to be normal. This condition is rare and tends to present at a young age. In the uncommon Lown-Ganong-Levine syndrome, accessory James fibres bypass the AV node and reach the bundle of His rather than directly stimulating the ventricular myocardium. Pre-excitation of the ventricles occurs resulting in a shortened PR interval on the ECG but no delta wave.

WPW syndrome occurs in 1 to 3 per 1000 people. It may be found in isolation or in association with a number of cardiac conditions including mitral valve prolapse and hypertrophic obstructive cardiomyopathy. False positive exercise tests often occur.

The accessory pathway is a strand of normal myocardium which results from incomplete separation of the atria and ventricles during embryological development. While the pathway can occur anywhere between the atria and ventricles, it most commonly lies on the left side of the heart (type A) and is associated with a positive complex in V1 on the ECG. A negative complex in V1 is seen in type B WPW where the accessory pathway is found on the right. ECG algorithms and complex electrophysiological techniques are used to define the exact location of the Kent bundle. Fibrosis of the accessory pathway may render it ineffective over time.

In sinus rhythm, atrial electrical activity is propagated along the accessory pathway at a greater velocity than through the AV node creating a short PR interval. The Kent bundle does not insert into the conducting system but into myocardium leading to premature activation of part of the ventricle and hence the delta wave. Conduction via the AV node soon catches up and depolarises the rest of the ventricle in the normal way.

Arrhythmias most commonly seen in WPW are atrial fibrillation (AF) and atrio-ventricular re-entry tachycardia (AVRT). Without the protection of the AV node, impulses from fibrillating atria can be transmitted directly to the ventricles via the Kent bundle resulting in a rapid ventricular response. Delta waves will be seen on the ECG. Acute heart failure and shock may ensue. The arrhythmia may deteriorate to ventricular fibrillation. Drugs such as digoxin and verapamil block the AV node and encourage conduction via the accessory and are contraindicated in WPW.

CHAPTER 4

Treatments include sotalol, flecainide, disopyramide, amioderone and electrical cardioversion. Internal cardioverter-defribillator (ICD) devices may be required.

The AV node remains refractory for a shorter period of time than the accessory pathway. Atrial ectopics can propagate through the AV node at a time before the accessory pathway has recovered. By the time the impulse reaches the ventricles, the accessory pathway has recovered and can transmit the impulse retrogradely towards the atria and then again down the AV node. A circus rhythm is set up leading to an AVRT. Ventricular ectopics can also trigger AVRTs. Delta waves are not seen in this condition.

Asymptomatic patients exposed to high risk situations (eg swimmers, climbers), high risk patients and those refractory to medical treatment may be candidates for destruction of the accessory pathway, usually by radio-frequency ablation.

By Dr R Thakkar

Reprinted with kind permission of *MIMS Cardiovascular*, July 2006

REFERENCES

[1] Pendleton D, Schofield T, Tate P and Havelock P *The New Consultation.* Oxford: Oxford University Press, 2003.

[2] Neighbour R. *The Inner Consultation: how to develop effective and intuitive consulting skills.* Lancaster: Kluwer Academic Press, 1987.

[3] Thakkar R. July 2006 Wolff-Parkinson-White syndrome in *MIMS Cardiovascular*, 1 (1): 46.

Chapter 5
Exam Circuit 1

CASE 1

Tip

✓ Start a stopwatch now and give yourself two minutes to read through the case notes and brainstorm any points you may want to bring up during the consultation.

INSTRUCTIONS TO CANDIDATE (CASE NOTES)

You are a new GP to the practice and have never met this patient before.

Name	Richard Harris
Age	59
Past medical history	MI and stent, 6 months ago
Current medication	Aspirin 75 mg od
	Clopidogrel 75 mg od
	Ramipril 5 mg od
	Simvastatin 40 mg nocte
	Atenolol 25 mg od
Social history	Married, two children
	Current smoker

Saw the practice nurse last week for blood pressure and routine blood tests:

Recent blood pressure:	120/80 mmHg
Recent blood test:	Hb 14.9 g/dl
	Total cholesterol 4.3 mmol/l
	HDL 1.7 mmol/l

BRAINSTORM

INSTRUCTIONS TO ROLE PLAYER (PATIENT)

NOT TO BE SEEN BY THE CANDIDATE

Opening statement:

'Hello Doctor, I've been breathless.'

Patient background:

You are Richard Harris, 59 years old.

You have recently gone back to work, as a foreman, after a heart attack 6 months ago. Once the doctors diagnosed your heart attack, they took you straight to a special unit where the cardiologists inserted a stent (tube-like structure) to hold open one of the arteries in your heart which was blocked.

You have been feeling breathless for about a year.

It is especially bad in the cold weather and when you exert yourself.

It is no worse at night than in the day time.

It is no worse laying flat in bed.

It is associated with a cough, productive of sputum which is sometimes green but never bloody. It tends to be productive for almost 6 months of the year.

The cough is not dry or tickly.

You don't get heart burn.

You sometimes wheeze with it.

There is no associated chest pain when you exert yourself. You don't experience palpitations.

You continue to smoke despite your recent heart attack.

You know you should give up but enjoy it; you are not ready to give up at the moment.

You would rather discuss your concerns about breathlessness than smoking.

You know that smoking causes lung cancer, but you don't know about the other diseases smoking is associated with.

> *You take your medications as prescribed.*
>
> *You did not take any medications prior to your heart attack. Your symptoms are no worse since starting the heart tablets.*
>
> *You are concerned you have lung cancer because you have smoked 20 a day since the age of 19. You have also been exposed to asbestos.*
>
> *You are happy in yourself and enjoy life.*
>
> Your twin girls are at university and your wife works as the local supermarket. There is no family history of asthma.

NOTES

DATA-GATHERING, TECHNICAL AND ASSESSMENT SKILLS

- This gentleman is experiencing breathlessness and it is important to establish the nature of the symptoms. By reminding yourself of the possible differential diagnosis of breathlessness a focused history should be intuitive.

- Causes of breathlessness relevant to this man include:

  - poor conditioning

  - cardiac: failure, arrhythmia, ischaemic heart disease: stent restenosis, de novo coronary lesions

  - respiratory: chronic obstructive pulmonary disease (COPD, this case), asthma, asbestosis, malignancy.

- Questions to consider include:

  - What does he mean by breathlessness?

- • what brings it on, moderate exertion, mild exertion, at rest, lying flat in bed? (Consider using the Medical Research Council (MRC) scale of breathlessness)

- • does he experience palpitations or exertional chest discomfort?

- Is it triggered by changes in temperature, season, stress, time of day? Does he cough or wheeze? Is the cough dry or productive?

- The patient continues to smoke which may point towards a cardiovascular or respiratory cause. Instructing him to stop smoking is counter-productive, particularly as he doesn't want to discuss smoking: respect his wishes. You may wish to ask him if he knows what the dangers of smoking are, but only if he is receptive to the discussion.

- If he did want to discuss smoking, consider the Cycle of Change of addiction:

The Cycle of Change was developed by psychologists Procheska and DeClimente[1]. It may be applied to any patient when managing a change in behaviour, and is likely to be relevant in the mock consultation. Take smoking: a patient who already smokes may thoroughly enjoy it, may be thinking about giving up or perhaps has planned a quit programme. This being the case, if a patient who is already keen to give up receives a lecture from their GP on the dangers of smoking, they may be frustrated with the care they receive from their GP. The GP may feel they have done their job but in reality, they have failed. Ascertaining what the patient's views are on smoking is a good way of gauging where they are in the cycle of change. That way, the patient can be helped and will feel listened to.

1. Precontemplation – patient enjoying behaviour, little motivation to change – eating too much, smoking etc. The doctor's role is to get the patient thinking that changing their behaviour would be in their health interests to do so. This may move the patient onto the contemplation stage.

2. Contemplation – patient is thinking they should give up their behaviour but haven't planned how to go about it.

3. Planning – active management plan to give up the behaviour. For example, smoking counselling, commence nicotine replacement, phased reduction in number of cigarettes smoked.

4. Action – quit date.

5. Maintenance – period of time patient abstains from behaviour.

6. Relapse – patient resumes behaviour, may enter cycle at stage 1, 2 or 3.

Reprinted from *GP ST: Stage 3 Assessment Handbook*.

*   He has smoked 20 packets a day for 40 years = 40-pack years.

*   The history points toward a diagnosis of COPD: he has a productive cough and wheeze without cardiac symptoms. If he had a dry cough, ramipril may be implicated. If he had wheeze without sputum production and his symptoms had started after he was commenced on cardiac drugs, atenolol may have been implicated in causing bronchospasm.

*   Examination of both the cardiovascular and respiratory systems is appropriate. Consider re-checking his blood pressure; 120/80 seems a bit too good to be true! The examiners will not be expecting an MRCGP-perfect systems-based examination; they will be more impressed if you perform a focused examination relevant to the patient. It would appropriate to examine him on the couch, top exposed if he is agreeable. Check his pulse, blood pressure, feel his cardiac apex, percuss for effusions and listen to his heart and breath sounds. Checking for conjunctival pallor is reasonable given he is breathless. Examination should be slick and shouldn't take long.

Tip

✓ **Practise your examination skills prior to the CSA until you are slick and efficient.**

CHAPTER 5

- Consider whether he has depression after his myocardial infarction and be sensitive when discussing the possibility of another chronic disease, eg COPD. Some data suggests 90% of patients with COPD have depression.

CLINICAL MANAGEMENT SKILLS

- Smoking cessation: most practices offer or have access to smoking cession clinics. He isn't keen to discuss smoking today but he may change his mind.

- His diagnosis is likely to be COPD, but you need to confirm the diagnosis. It is important to refer him to the practice nurse for spirometry. Most practices will have a spirometer; given that the Quality and Outcomes Framework (QOF) rewards its use. Reversibility resting is included in the 2008/2009 QOF in order to exclude asthma.

- Given his exposure to cigarette smoke as well as asbestos, it would be reasonable to organise a chest radiograph.

- Organising a full blood count may be appropriate as he is breathless, to ensure he is not anaemic, particularly as he is on aspirin and clopidogrel.

INTERPERSONAL SKILLS

- Breathlessness is a frightening experience. It is important to make him feel at ease and free to express his fears.

- Remember, until he has had formal spirometry, it wouldn't be wise to give him a formal diagnosis of COPD. You may however, introduce the idea of him having a smoking related disease. How would you do this? You may ask if knows anyone else with smoking related lung problems.

- Offer to discuss smoking if he so wishes; be explicit, Discuss it without being patronising, but only if he wishes to do so. By explaining the risks of smoking, you may encourage him to give up. He may want to attend a smoking cessation clinic. Would he prefer nicotine replacement therapy or alternative treatments rather than attend a dedicated clinic? If he doesn't want to use the clinic, why not, what are his fears? He may ask about a new drug he has read about in the papers: Champix® (varenicline).

- How will you explain what COPD is? Perhaps use visual aids or suggest he looks at a website such as www.patient.co.uk

- What are his concerns? This patient is concerned about lung cancer and has little idea about COPD. How can you reassure him; how would he like to be reassured: a chest radiograph for example?

- Once a discussion has taken place about the possibility of COPD, negotiate whether he is happy to have appropriate investigations. He may not want to; perhaps he would rather have a chest radiograph, perhaps give up smoking and then see if his symptoms improve.

- Does he know what spirometry is?

- He may ask about treatment of COPD, despite not having confirmatory tests as yet. If you are running out of time it is appropriate to apologise and suggest, if he wouldn't mind, talking through the treatment if the diagnosis is confirmed.

- Appropriate follow-up is required to provide further encouragement in smoking cessation and to follow up results of investigations and to formulate any treatment strategies.

- Safety-netting is required to seek advice if he becomes acutely breathless.

SMOKING CESSATION TREATMENT OPTIONS

	BUPROPRION	NICOTINE	VARENICLINE
BRAND	Zyban	Nicorette Nicotinell Niquitin Niquitin CQ	Champix
PRESENTATION	Prolonged release, film-coated tablets	Gum Inhalator (Nicorette only) Lozenges Microtabs (Nicorette only) Nasal spray (Nicorette only) Transdermal patches	Film-coated tablets
TREATMENT DURATION	7–9 weeks	10–12 weeks	12 weeks
CONTRAINDICATIONS	• History of seizures • CNS tumour • Bulimia, anorexia nervosa • Bipolar disorder • Severe hepatic cirrhosis • Patients experiencing abrupt withdrawal of alcohol or benzodiazepines	None	None
USE IN PREGNANCY	No	Yes • Intermittent dosing products are preferable as they provide lower daily dose of nicotine • Patches may be preferred if woman suffering from nausea • Patches should be removed before going to bed • Aim to discontinue after 2–3 months	No
USE IN LACTATION	No	Yes • Intermittent dosing products are preferable	No
RECOMMENDED BY NICE	Yes	Yes	Yes
MODE OF ACTION	Inhibits the reuptake of noradrenaline and dopamine resulting in a reduction in craving and withdrawal symptoms.	Nicotine replacement therapy allows the psychological addition of the smoking habit to be dealt with separately from the physical addiction to nicotine.	Blinds nicotine acetylcholine receptors to alleviate symptoms of craving and withdrawal. Also competes with nicotine at the receptor binding sites, resulting in a reduction of the rewarding and reinforcing effects of smoking.

• All smokers should be advised to stop and offered help if interested in doing so.

• Smoking cessation therapies should be offered when appropriate, and where possible, smokers should have access to a smoking cessation clinic or programme for behavioural support.

Fig. 7 Smoking cessation treatment options

Reproduced with the kind permission of MIMS

CHAPTER 5

NOTES ON COPD

GUIDELINES PUBLISHED BY THE NATIONAL INSTITUTE FOR HEALTH AND CLINICAL EXCELLENCE (NICE), 2004

- Consider diagnosis in:
    - those over 35 years old who are current smokers or ex-smokers
    - those with a history of chronic cough, wheeze, regular sputum production and exertional breathlessness
    - those who have bronchitis occurring frequently in winter.
- COPD likely if FEV_1 < 80% predicted and FEV_1/FVC < 0.7
- Mild COPD: FEV_1 50–80% of predicted
- Moderate COPD: FEV_1 30–50% of predicted
- Severe COPD: FEV_1 < 30% of predicted
- Consider asthma if > 400 ml (FEV_1) response to bronchodilators/prednisolone trial
- All patients should be educated: smoking cessation advice; influenza vaccination
- Mild disease: short acting β-agonists, anti-cholinergic or combination – use long acting drug if required
- Moderate/Severe: long acting β-agonists and anti-cholinergics: trial of inhaled corticosteroids (discontinue if no effect after 4 weeks use)
- Consider pulmonary rehabilitation for MRC grade 3–5.

CASE 2

INSTRUCTIONS TO CANDIDATES (CASE NOTES)

Name   Rose Shanahan

Age   61

Past medical history   Osteoarthritis

Total knee replacement: 3 weeks ago

Hypertension

Current medication   Cocodamol 30/500 max 2 qds

Amlodipine 5mg od

Social history   Lives with husband

Saw the practice nurse this morning for blood pressure and routine blood tests:

Blood pressure this am   136/78 mmHg

BRAINSTORM

INSTRUCTIONS TO ROLE PLAYER (PATIENT)

NOT TO BE SEEN BY THE CANDIDATE

Opening statement:

'Hi Doctor, I want a second opinion.'

Patient background:

You are Rose Shanahan, you are 61 years old.

You had a total knee replacement of your right knee 3 weeks ago.

You are not happy with it and would like a second opinion to see if it was done properly.

It is still painful.

You were expecting it to be pain free by now.

You can't remember exactly what the surgeon and physiotherapist told you about recovery.

You are keen to get back to dancing.

It has been warm and swollen since the operation. The swelling is less than it was last week.

You have not felt feverish.

The wound is looking clean and it hasn't oozed any pus.

Admittedly it has been getting less painful as time goes by.

You want to drive; it is important as you have a disabled grandchild who needs to be taken to his therapy group while your daughter is at work.

You don't like pills and only take 1 cocodamol (30/500) tablet at night.

You're embarrassed to say that the cocodamol made you constipated, you have not suffered any weight loss or gain, and you have never seen any blood in the stool.

You have never had a stomach ulcer and have never had problems with ibuprofen. You are not asthmatic.

NOTES

DATA-GATHERING, TECHNICAL AND ASSESSMENT SKILLS

- Establishing what the patient was told by the hospital is important.

- Was she given any leaflets by the hospital and has she read them?

- You should ask about and examine to exclude complications of knee replacement, eg features of deep vein thrombosis (DVT), infection, peroneal nerve palsy, vascular complications.

- Has she tried to drive so far?

- What analgesia is she taking?

- Does she have any side effects from her medication; does she know what side effects she may expect?

- Perhaps consider other causes of constipation; does she have any features of hypothyroidism, has she noticed any red flag symptoms suggestive of bowel cancer?

CLINICAL MANAGEMENT SKILLS

- Offer alternative analgesia.

- Offer laxatives.

- Consider full blood count (FBC) and C-reactive protein (CRP) if concerned about infection. If you have a high index of suspicion for infection or DVT, she should be referred to secondary care for assessment.

INTERPERSONAL SKILLS

- This consultation is partly about managing the patient's expectations.

- Does she know how long it takes most people to recover? Swimming can commence once the wound has healed. Non-stressful activities, including dancing, can commence around 6 weeks whereas activities that stress the joint should be avoided, eg squash.

- Does she know anyone else who may have had a knee replacement; how long did they take to fully recover? In general, patients may take 2 months before they return to work.

- What does she hope another surgeon would do at this early stage?

- Does she have any particular concerns that you may be able to address?

- Try to get her to realise why driving may be dangerous, perhaps by asking her if she knows what the risks are. If she can't see why driving may be dangerous, perhaps offer an example, eg inability to perform an emergency stop. Driving may commence as soon as 1 week after left knee replacement but may be 4–6 weeks after right knee replacement.

- Explore why she is not keen to take her analgesia. Can you offer her options (eg paracetamol, non-steroidal anti-inflammatory drugs (NSAIDS)) and agree a plan that suits her. You will need to discuss the pros and cons of each option so she can make an informed choice.

- Reiterate the complications of having knee replacement, and check you understand her and she understands you.

- Share a management plan together and agree a reasonable follow-up appointment.

Detailed notes on 'Knee Joint Replacements – What a GP Needs to Know' are produced by www.patient.co.uk.

CHAPTER 5

CASE 3

INSTRUCTIONS TO CANDIDATES (CASE NOTES)

Name   Sarah Jones

Date of birth (age) 59

The patient is new to the surgery and her notes have not been summarised onto the computer records.

BRAINSTORM

Tip

✓ In the examination, there may be cases where you have little information to brainstorm points you would like to bring up. If so, look at future cases or take a breather and compose yourself.

INSTRUCTIONS TO ROLE PLAYER (PATIENT)

NOT TO BE SEEN BY THE CANDIDATE

Opening statement:

'Hello, I was wondering if I could have some more of my tablets' (you have an empty box of your old tablets).

Patient background:

Your name is Sarah Jones, you are 59 yeas old.

You are a headmistress and have recently moved to the local area.

You live with your husband and don't have children (through choice).

You are very embarrassed about why you've come to see the doctor today.

The main reason for you coming is vaginal bleeding.

You first ask for a repeat prescription of your blood pressure tablets (amlodipine 5 mg) which you've been on for 2 years. Your blood pressure has always been well controlled on this drug and you only had it checked last week by your old GP who said it was 135/70.

You have never smoked and have a very healthy diet.

You exercise regularly.

Your GP recently checked your cholesterol which was excellent but you can't remember the number.

He also checked to see if you were diabetic, which you're not.

Both your parents had strokes in their 80s.

CHAPTER 5

Your mother also had endometrial (womb) cancer.

You appear distracted and when prompted, you allude (through non-verbal cues) to their being something else you would like to discuss; something 'embarrassing'. If the doctor doesn't ask if there is something worrying you, you admit there is something embarrassing you'd like to discuss. You do this early in the consultation.

You have experienced vaginal spotting (fresh blood) for 4 months.

It has been getting heavier lately and you are now bleeding on a daily basis.

Your best friend urged you to see the doctor.

You sometimes pass blood clots.

You're sexually active and faithful to your partner.

Bleeding isn't provoked by intercourse.

You don't have any pelvic pain.

Your last smear, 2 years ago, was normal.

You had the menopause at age 53.

You have felt more tired lately.

You have been frightened in case you have womb cancer, as your mother had.

You have not been experiencing bloating or breathlessness.

You do not want an intimate examination today.

You would like to be referred to a female gynaecologist for further investigation.

You are otherwise well and have never had any other medical problems.

CHAPTER 5

NOTES

DATA-GATHERING, TECHNICAL AND ASSESSMENT SKILLS

- It is important to take a brief history regarding high blood pressure. How long has she had it for? Does she have any other cardiovascular risk factors? It is sometimes difficult to take over the care of a chronic disease in a new patient. In some situations, there may be good reason to double-check the patient's blood pressure again. In this case it is useful to have her blood pressure on your record, especially if you are responsible for the drug you are going to prescribe. In addition, this will satisfy the QOF requirement.

- Postmenopausal bleeding (PMB) should be taken seriously as it may be a sign of malignancy.

- It is generally accepted that bleeding 12 months after the last menstrual period is considered postmenopausal.

- Ten percent of women with PMB will have endometrial carcinoma. It is important to consider when the bleeding started, the approximate volume of blood loss, and when it happens. Smear history is relevant in case the bleeding is cervical in origin.

- Risk factors for endometrial carcinoma should be part of the history and includes; age (peak age approx 60), obesity, parity (higher incidence in nulliparous women), late menopause, diabetes, unopposed oestrogen (which is why hormone replacement therapy (HRT) should include cyclical progestogen in women who have not had a hysterectomy), and family history (including a family history of hereditary non-polyposis colorectal cancer). In premenopausal women, irregular or heavy periods may be the presenting feature.

- Tamoxifen increases the risk of endometrial carcinoma.

CHAPTER 5

- HRT complicates the clinical picture. If patients are on HRT, bleeding may also be caused by poor compliance or poor absorption. One should enquire if the bleeding is cyclical and if they are taking other medications (which can interact).

- Clinical examination is not always necessary and this is stated in the Scottish Intercollegiate Guidelines Network (SIGN) guidelines.

- Examination of the abdomen wouldn't be unreasonable to check for a bulky uterus and evidence of metastatic disease. You may want to offer an abdominal examination, justifying your reasoning, as long as she is agreeable.

Tip

✓ **For the purposes of this examination, intimate examinations are not permitted. However, you should express to the examiner that you would consider performing such an examination and why.**

- Her tiredness is likely to be secondary to anaemia. It would be reasonable to consider whether anaemia has caused cardio-respiratory compromise.

CLINICAL MANAGEMENT SKILLS

- She should be given a repeat prescription for amlodipine and arrange follow-up.

- This patient may have a gynaecological malignancy. She has a number of risk factors for endometrial cancer and she should be referred to the gynaecology team on a 2 week wait (2WW) basis.

- She is feeling tired and it is likely the bleeding has lead to anaemia. Organising a full blood count is entirely appropriate.

CHAPTER 5

INTERPERSONAL SKILLS

- PMB is a clearly a sensitive issue for her and one should be aware of this.

- She is obviously embarrassed; make her feel at ease. Non-verbal cues may be used, for example: 'You look very worried…you seem to have something on your mind…are you ok? You seem troubled…'

- Check that you understand exactly what the history is, perhaps by summarising the history back to her.

- Consider what her fears are: cancer (given her mother had endometrial cancer too). If you are aware what her fears are, she will be satisfied you are taking them into account in your management.

- Introducing the idea that PMB may have a sinister aetiology is required to agree a management plan. This must be done in a sensitive manner, perhaps by asking her what she thinks may be the cause of the bleeding, how her mum presented, or what her concerns are. In this way, the discussion can be based around her own health beliefs.

- A management plan should be agreed by you both (shared management).

- She should be appropriately followed up; to ensure she has had her blood tests and to discuss the results with her, to ensure she has received an appointment from the gynaecologist, and that she has indeed attended. She may also want to come back in case she has more questions; she should know this opportunity is available.

CASE 4

INSTRUCTIONS TO CANDIDATES (CASE NOTES)

Name	Petra Lipinski
Age	62
Past medical history	Appendicectomy, 2001
	Hypertension
	Osteoarthritis, knees
Current medication	Ramipril 5 mg od
	Cocodamol, 30/500 max 2 qds
Allergies	NSAIDS
	Amlodipine
Social history	Lives with partner
	Language teacher

Last consultation (2 months ago):

BP 123/80

BMI 22

Left knee pain continues – not locking; injected with 80 mg methylprednisolone, aseptic technique. Medial approach. Warned re infections. Review if concerned; otherwise repeat injection in 6 months.

CHAPTER 5

69

BRAINSTORM

INSTRUCTIONS TO ROLE PLAYER (PATIENT)

NOT TO BE SEEN BY THE CANDIDATE

Opening statement:

'My knee is playing up again doctor'

Patient background:

You are Petra Lipinski, a 62-year-old teacher.

You have been in the UK for 30 years.

You have had high blood pressure for 10 years which has always been well controlled on ramipril.

You have osteoarthritis in both knees *from your days as a runner.*

Your arthritis was formally diagnosed 15 years ago by X-ray.

Your left knee has always been the one that has caused you the most pain.

You're aware the X-ray of the left knee revealed more advanced arthritis than the right.

Your right knee has never caused you any problems.

You can't quite remember exactly what osteoarthritis is. You think it is when the joints get damaged.

You take cocodamol 30/500, 2 tablets, four times a day to help with pain in your left knee.

You buy lactulose syrup to help with constipation, which you always get with codeine.

You can't take any drugs like ibuprofen, they all cause a rash.

You have steroid injections twice a year to help with the pain.

The injections normally help but your knee has become painful only 2 months after your previous injection.

You don't exercise and have never tried physiotherapy or acupuncture.

You have never tried glucosamine, although you have heard of it.

CHAPTER 5

71

The knee doesn't give way or lock.

It is impacting on your quality of life and causes you pain on a daily basis, especially whenever you are on your feet.

You are often in pain at work and sometimes have to teach sitting down. Your headmaster doesn't mind and he is very supportive.

You find the pain distracting during lesson times.

You are able to wash and dress yourself.

Stairs can be painful and you sometimes have to take short steps to reduce the pain.

All of your other joints are fine.

You are not unhappy in yourself.

You are keen to try physiotherapy and swimming.

You would rather not have stronger pain killers at this stage.

You would consider taking glucosamine, but you're not sure where to get it from.

You are not keen on acupuncture.

You don't want to be referred to an orthopaedic surgeon; you are fearful of having a knee replacement. You know someone who recently had a replacement and they are in constant pain.

You're happy to try out some of the therapies discussed and review the situation in a few months.

NOTES

NICE published guidelines on osteoarthritis in February 2008. The important points have been incorporated into these notes.

DATA-GATHERING, TECHNICAL AND ASSESSMENT SKILLS

- Important features to consider with knee pain include:
  - the background to the condition – when was it diagnosed, how did she get it (eg running – as in this case, sport, accident, septic joint)
  - are other joints are affected?
  - treatment so far? – drugs (over the counter and prescribed), physiotherapy, acupuncture, joint injection with steroid
  - treatments that have worked
  - impact on her quality of life – home and work
  - is it making her unhappy?
  - does the knee give way or lock? If so, under what circumstances?
- Examination of the knee should ideally be done on the couch. Remember – look, feel, move, function. You should look for deformity and scars, palpate for joint-line tenderness and crepitus, assess range of movement, and check for laxity of the collateral and cruciate ligaments. Asking her to walk may reveal an antalgic gait.

CLINICAL MANAGEMENT SKILLS

- Consider:
  - holistic approach
  - educate patient on osteoarthritis (OA)
  - encourage exercise

CHAPTER 5

- sensible footwear

- heat/cold packs

- transcutaneous electrical nerve stimulation (TENS) machine

- analgesia

- topical capsaicin

- intra-articular steroid injections

- physiotherapy/occupational therapy

- glucosamine not advised by NICE – however, Gait trial, 2006, showed statistically significant benefit

- referral for arthroscopic lavage/debridement shouldn't be offered unless knee locking

- referral for surgery if symptoms have substantial impact on quality of life and if non-surgical treatments have failed.

INTERPERSONAL SKILLS

- Consider what the patient's thoughts are; does she know what osteoarthritis actually is?

- Is she aware how she may have developed it?

- What are her concerns? eg knee replacement, disability.

- What are her expectations? What does she hope to achieve from treatments? Does she know what the side effects may be?

- Share management options, let her know what options are available to her, giving pros and cons and help her choose a strategy that is acceptable to her.

- Agree suitable follow-up.

CASE 5

INSTRUCTIONS TO CANDIDATES (CASE NOTES)

Name	Mr Rizwan Patel
Occupation	Economics teacher
Age	51
Past medical history	Obesity
	Hypercholesterolaemia
Current medication	Atorvastatin 40 mg nocte
Family History	Father MI
	Mother CVA
Social History	Originally from South Asia
	Married, three children

Saw the practice nurse last week for blood pressure and routine blood tests:

Recent blood pressures
(taken on three separate occasions by the nurse)

175/93, 172/97, 165/96 mmHg

Recent blood tests	Total cholesterol 4.8 mmol/l
	HDL 0.9 mmol/l
	eGFR > 90 ml/min

BRAINSTORM

INSTRUCTIONS TO ROLE PLAYER (PATIENT)

NOT TO BE SEEN BY THE CANDIDATE

Opening statement:

'Hello Doctor! I've been told to see you by the nurse. My blood pressure is too high!'

Patient background:

Your name is Rizwan Patel, you are 51 years old.

You have been seeing the practice nurse over the past month for blood pressure (BP) checks. It has been consistently high and she has asked you to see the doctor.

You have a history of high cholesterol which runs in your family. You take a cholesterol tablet for this (atorvastatin 40 mg).

You take your medication every day without fail.

You are not quite sure what blood pressure means, in particular you would like to know what the ideal BP is and what the significance of each number is.

You are unsure why treating blood pressure is important, although you are willing to take any medication the doctor suggests.

You drink 2 × 250 ml glasses of (12%) wine per night. You sometimes don't drink any alcohol at all, but two glasses is the norm. You never drink in the mornings. Last week, you went away for a city break and didn't drink at all.

You don't exercise although you know you should.

When you do exert yourself you do not experience any chest discomfort.

You are overweight and don't look after your diet.

You have never smoked.

You don't have to get up in the night to pass urine and don't complain of excessive thirst or tiredness.

You wonder what you can do to reduce your blood pressure yourself. You don't mind taking tablets in the meantime until you can alter your lifestyle.

NOTES

DATA-GATHERING, TECHNICAL AND ASSESSMENT SKILLS

- This patient is at risk of cardiovascular disease because of his ethnicity, hypertension requirement to take statins, and obesity.

- His blood pressure should be rechecked in order to confirm that it is high. (The examiner may tell you what today's reading is.)

- It is important to consider risk factors for hypertension; these include obesity and alcohol. His weight should be measured.

- For the examination, weighing him without shoes and debris in his pockets is sufficient. You may say to him that you will document that he was weighed with his clothes on but without shoes.

- His weekly alcohol consumption should be calculated using his daily consumption:

    - (ml)/1000 × % alcohol = 500/1000 × 12 = 6 units.

    - Therefore his weekly consumption is: 6 × 7 = 42 units.

- One should sensitively establish whether he is dependant on alcohol.

- Salt and fat consumption should also be noted.

- Other cardiovascular risk factors should be discussed and checked, including smoking status and family history.

- It would be prudent to establish whether is has symptoms suggestive of coronary artery disease: exertional chest pain and breathlessness.

- A cardiovascular examination is important, in part, to establish whether there are any signs of aortic stenosis if you are considering prescribing ACE-inhibitors (ACE-I).

Tip

✓ You should not expect to find any abnormal signs during the CSA. If you do, it is likely to be by chance.

- This patient may be diabetic and you should ask about symptoms suggestive of hyperglycaemia.

CLINICAL MANAGEMENT SKILLS

- A discussion about lifestyle should take place.

- Advise that addressing his lifestyle issues may eliminate the need for blood pressure medication which may provide an added incentive to lose weight and reduce his alcohol intake.

- According to the cycle of change of addiction, if he already realises he wants to address lifestyle issues, your time is better spent discussing how he can reduce his weight and alcohol consumption. Of course, if he is resistant to this perhaps discussing the risks of not addressing lifestyle and the benefits of doing so would be appropriate.

- Ideally he should cut down on alcohol, improve his diet and exercise more.

- He should be encouraged to loose around 1–2 lbs (approx 0.5–1 kg)/ week of weight by diet and exercise. This could be monitored by the practice health care assistant (HCA).

- Given his consistently high blood pressure, he ought to be started on medication as per the joint British Hypertension Society/NICE guidelines. As he is under the age of 55 he should be commenced on an ACE-I. He should be warned about the side effects – as detailed in the British National Formulary (BNF) – including first dose hypotension, cough and angio-oedema.

- His creatinine should be monitored around 10 days after commencement of an ACE-I (explain why). After his blood test, you should review him to discuss the result and recheck his blood pressure. If his blood pressure is not controlled the dose could be increased and his creatinine rechecked accordingly.

CHAPTER 5

- He should be warned that he may need higher doses of the drug and more than one drug may be required (he will therefore know what to expect).

Tip

✓ **Don't be reluctant to use your BNF in the CSA. The examination may be considered as a driving test. You have to demonstrate you're a good doctor.**

- His blood glucose should be checked.

INTERPERSONAL SKILLS

- Discussing a patient's lifestyle, including weight and alcohol consumption, is not always easy and it should be done sensitively. One way around this would be to ask him about what he thinks about his own lifestyle and the effects it may have on his health (his ideas). If prompting is required, you could give some of the factors which contribute to high blood pressure; include alcohol and being overweight. He may then offer his sentiments regarding both of these.

- What are his ideas on the causes of cardiovascular disease?

- It is important to get him on board with lifestyle changes.

- Education and regular follow-up are both important in this case. He has a number of questions and he should be given the opportunity to ask these and any concerns that he has.

- Managing his expectations may improve his adherence to medication and maintain his satisfaction. Many patients don't realise they may have to stay on blood pressure medication permanently (around 70% of patients will remain on anti-hypertensive drugs), and few realise the initial dose may not be sufficient to control it. Explain he may need to go on higher dose medication and more than one drug if the initial dose you prescribed doesn't control his blood pressure.

- Without explanation, patients may think they only need to take a one month course as prescribed.

CHAPTER 5

MANAGEMENT OF HYPERTENSION IN ADULTS IN PRIMARY CARE NICE GUIDELINE

Measurement

- Use an average of two seated BP readings from at least two visits to guide the decision to treat.
- Take a standing reading in patients with symptoms of postural hypotension.
- Measure BP on both of patient's arms with higher value identifying the reference arm for future measurement.
- Test for proteinuria. Measure plasma glucose, electrolytes, creatinine, serum total cholesterol and HDL-cholesterol. Arrange as 12-lead ECG.
- Estimate 10-year cardiovascular disease (CVD) risk in accordance with the Joint British Societies assessment scheme www.bhsoc.org.

Note: Routine use of automated ambulatory BP monitoring or home monitoring devices in primary care is not currently recommended.

Aims

- To reduce diastolic BP to ≤90 mmHg.
- To reduce systolic BP to ≤140 mmHg.

Note: Screening for hypertension, management of hypertension in pregnancy and specialist management of secondary hypertension are not addressed by the NICE guideline. Patients with existing coronary heart disease (CHD) or diabetes should be managed in line with current national guidance for these conditions.

BP (mmHg)	Major Risk Factors	Recommended Action
		Offer lifestyle advice initially and then periodically to all patients.
>140/90	–	Reassess in 5 years.
>140/90	–	Remeasure at min. of two subsequent clinics (at monthly intervals or more frequently in case of more severe hypertension). If raised BP persists in patients without established cardiovascular disease, the need for formal assessment of cardiovascular disease, the need for formal assessment of cardiovascular risk should be discussed. Reassess in 1 year.
>140/90	+	Offer drug therapy to patients with raised cardiovascular risk (10-year risk of CVD ≥20% or existing cardiovascular disease or target organ damage) with BP persistently >140/90 mmHg.
≥160/100	+/–	Offer drug therapy to patients with high BP persistently ≥160/100 mmHg.

Non-pharmacological measures

- Assess patients' diet and exercise patterns and encourage appropriate lifestyle changes.
- Advise patients to:
    - Limit weekly alcohol intake
    - Avoid excessive consumption of coffee (≥5 cups/day) and other caffeine-rich products.
    - Limit dietary sodium intake (≥6 g/day) by reducing intake or substituting sodium salt.
- Offer smoking cessation help and advice.
- Encourage stress reduction.

Note: Calcium, magnesium or potassium supplements should not be offered as a method for reducing BP.

Treatment

- Offer treatment as described below to all patients regardless of age and ethnicity – be prepared to tailor drug therapy for individuals who do not respond to the sequence of drugs indicated.
- Offer patients over 80 years the same treatment as younger patients taking account of any co-morbidity and patient's existing burden of drug use.
- Offer patients with isolated systolic hypertension (systolic BP>160mmHg) the same treatment as patients with both raised systolic and diastolic BP.
- Provide patients with appropriate guidance and material about the benefits of drugs and the unwanted side-effects that may occur in other to help patients make informed choices.
- Where possible, recommend treatment with drugs that can be taken once daily.
- Prescribe generic preparations where these are appropriate and minimise cost.

CHAPTER 5

TREATMENT ALGORITHM

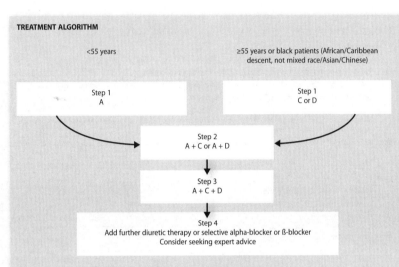

A = ACE inhibitor (or angiotensin II receptor antagonist if ACE inhibitor not tolerated)
C = Calcium antagonist
D = Thiazide-type diuretic

Note

– *ß-blockers are not a preferred initial therapy but are an alternative in patients <55 years with an intolerance or contraindication to ACE inhibitors (or angiotensin II receptor antagonists) including women of childbearing potential.*

– *In patients well controlled with a regimen that includes a ß-blocker there is no absolute need to replace the ß-blocker with an alternative agent.*

– *If therapy initiated with a ß-blocker, add a calcium antagonist rather than a thiazide-type diuretic to reduce risk of diabetes.*

Follow-up

• Annual review – monitor BP, provide patients with support and discuss lifestyle, symptoms and medication.

• Offer patients who are motivated to make lifestyle changes, want to stop using antihypertensives and who are at low cardiovascular risk and have well controlled BP a trial reduction or withdrawal of therapy with appropriate lifestyle guidance and ongoing review.

Specialist referral

• Consider in patients with signs and symptoms suggesting secondary cause of hypertension. Accelerated (malignant) hypertension and suspected phaeochromocytoma require immediate referral.

• Consider in patients with symptoms of, or documented postural hypotension (fall in systolic BP when standing of 20 mmHg or more).

• Consider in patients with unusual signs or symptoms or in those whose management depends critically on the accurate measurement of their BP.

Adapted from: NICE Clinical Guideline 34 (July 2006) – Hypertension: management of hypertension in adults in primary care (primary update of NICE Clinical Guideline 18). The full NICE guideline is available at www.nice.org.uk. A quick reference guide is also available.

Fig. 8 Management of hypertension in adults in Primary Care, Nice guidelines

Reproduced with the kind permission of MIMS

CHAPTER 5

ACE INHIBITORS AND RENAL ARTERY STENOSIS[2]

Renal artery stenosis, quite simply, describes narrowing of the renal artery or arteries depending whether it is uni- or bilateral. Epidemiology varies widely depending on the literature and its true incidence is not known.

There are essentially two likely pathological processes at work – atherosclerosis and fibromuscular dysplasia. Atherosclerosis accounts for approximately 70-90 per cent of renal artery stenosis and tends to occur in men over the age of 50.

Risk factors are similar to those for cardiovascular disease and it is no surprise that there is considerable overlap between the two conditions as well as with other vasculopathies. Up to 5 per cent of hypertensive patients may have renovascular disease. Atherosclerotic renal artery stenosis increases mortality risk in those undergoing cardiac catheterisation.

The remainder of renal artery stenosis cases are caused by fibromuscular dysplasia, which is seen more frequently in younger females. In this condition, stenosis is bilateral in 60 per cent of cases and, unlike vascular renal artery stenosis, tends to occur in mid and distal renal arteries. Total arterial occlusion is rare, unlike in atherosclerotic disease where 15 per cent of cases go on to occlude.

PRESENTATION AND MANAGEMENT

Except for ACE inhibitor-induced reduction in renal function, renal artery stenosis may present with resistant hypertension (the majority of hypertension in these patients is not renovascular in origin), pulmonary oedema, renal failure (with or without hypertension), or clinically in vasculopaths or those with abdominal bruits.

Proteinuria, below nephrotic range, may be the only presenting feature. Diagnostic techniques vary and include captopril stimulation tests, ACE inhibitor renography, duplex ultrasound, CT, MRI and angiography. Duplex ultrasound, in the right hands, has a 98 per cent specificity and sensitivity. Conventional ultrasound scanning may demonstrate shrunken (<8 cm) kidneys.

CHAPTER 5

83

The jury is still out on the optimal treatment modality for renal artery stenosis. One study demonstrated a 30.6 per cent cure rate and 61.1 per cent improvement in blood pressure (BP) using surgical techniques.

Thrombosis and re-stenosis may affect around 4 per cent of patients. Percutaneous intervention has superseded open surgery and long term outcome studies have shown little difference between the two groups. Stents dramatically reduce re-stenosis rates.

All patients with atherosclerotic renal artery stenosis should have their vascular risk factors managed. Smoking cessation, diet and exercise advice should be given; BP, cholesterol and diabetes should all be monitored and controlled. Anti-platelet agents should be prescribed and calcium channel blockers may be used as an effective alternative for BP control. Clearly, ACE inhibitors should be used with caution.

THE BENEFITS AND RISKS OF ACE INHIBITORS

ACE inhibitors were developed in the 1970s and have revolutionised modern medical practice. Optimised management of MI, cardiac failure, hypertension and proteinuria all require the use of ACE inhibitors in addition to other treatments.

Several high quality studies have demonstrated a significant reduction in cardiovascular morbidity and mortality when these drugs are used. Unfortunately, as with most drugs, there are side-effects and contraindications (including significant aortic stenosis and renal artery stenosis).

First-dose hypotension may be particularly marked in those who are already volume depleted, for example those taking diuretics. A dry irritating cough, caused by elevated pulmonary bradykinin, is more commonly seen in women and can affect up to one in five patients. As the cough may be particularly troublesome at night, obstructive airways disease should be excluded.

Voice changes, taste alteration, angioedema, abdominal pain, rash, blood dyscrasias and hyperkalaemia are all seen. A reduction in blood glucose is a well documented side-effect and ACE inhibitors may account for nearly 14 per cent of hypoglycaemia-related hospital admissions.

While ACE inhibitors have been shown to be effective in certain kidney disorders, there are conditions such as renal artery stenosis where they, and angiotensin receptor blockers (ARBs), may adversely affect renal function.

Other conditions that predispose to acute renal failure with ACE inhibitors include chronic renal diseases such as polycystic kidney disease, cardiac failure, hypovolaemia and cirrhosis. ACE inhibitors may also cause renal tubular acidosis and possibly, renal artery thrombosis.

HOW ACE INHIBITORS WORK

As the name suggests, ACE inhibitors suppress the activity of ACE, an enzyme central to the renin-angiotensin-aldosterone (RAS) system. The production of renin, an enzyme stored in the juxtaglomerular apparatus, is stimulated by a reduction in renal perfusion, such as occurs in renal artery stenosis or low blood pressure (including iatrogenic), changes in sodium concentration, prostaglandin changes and neurohormonal sympathetic stimulation.

Once released into the circulation, renin cleaves angiotensinogen to form the biologically inactive angiotensin I. ACE then cleaves two more amino acids to form angiotensin II, a process that occurs primarily in the lungs.

ACE is also involved in the breakdown of bradykinin. Angiotensin II stimulates the adrenal cortex to produce aldosterone. It is a powerful biological vasoconstrictor.

Angiotensin II forms part of the renal autoregulation of glomerular perfusion mechanism. The afferent (pre-glomerular) arteriolar tone is reduced in cases where renal perfusion falls, thereby increasing glomerular blood flow and maintaining glomerular filtration. If this response is inadequate renin is released, activating the RAS cascade, leading to angiotensin II mediated constriction of the efferent (post-glomerular) arteriole. Pressure within the glomerulus is therefore increased and filtration restored.

RENAL ARTERY STENOSIS AND ACE INHIBITORS

In renal artery stenosis the afferent pressure is reduced by the narrowed vessel; hence autoregulation is almost exclusively dependant on changes in efferent arteriolar tone. As ACE inhibitors interfere with the production

CHAPTER 5

of angiotensin II, autoregulation is impaired, glomerular perfusion falls, renal ischaemic nephropathy develops and renal failure ensues.

ACE inhibitors are very effective when treating renovascular hypertension, especially in combination with diuretics, as long as there is no significant deterioration in GFR. Prior to commencing a patient on an ACE inhibitor, it is recommended that renal function and potassium are checked. If creatinine exceeds 150 micromol/l, NICE recommends that these drugs should only be introduced under specialist supervision.

Care should be particularly taken in at risk groups including those with known vascular disease and patients on diuretics or antihypertensives who may be on the verge of renal hypoperfusion. In severe bilateral renal artery stenosis, any antihypertensive may reduce renal artery perfusion.

Bloods should be rechecked soon after starting ACE inhibitors and after each dose increase. Patients should be started at the lowest dose and up-titrated as far as they are tolerated or the desired effect is achieved.

Up to half of people with bilateral renal artery stenosis will have a mild decline in GFR although other renal diseases may behave in a similar way. A mild increase in creatinine is acceptable and may demonstrate efficacy of ACE inhibitors according to some recent reports.

Around 5–10 per cent of patients will endure a significant reduction in GFR. A 30 per cent or greater rise in creatinine or a 20 per cent fall in GFR is suspicious and referral for further investigation should be considered along with stopping the ACE inhibitor/ARB. Renal artery stenosis often presents this way.

In patients who have critical artery stenosis, ACE inhibitors may precipitate acute renal failure requiring urgent intervention. In the context of chronic heart failure, NICE suggests that a 50 per cent rise in creatinine above pre-ACE inhibitor levels or an increase to 200 micromol/L may be acceptable.

By Dr Raj Thakkar

Reproduced with kind permission of MIMS Cardiovascular, pending publication 2008

FURTHER READING

BHF Fact file 07/2002. ACE-inhibitors: an update. www.bhf.org.uk/factfiles

Greenan M, Dworkin L (2006). Renal artery stenosis. *Nephrol Rounds* 4(4): 1–6.

Haller C (2002).Arteriosclerotic renal artery stenosis: conservative versus interventional management. *Heart* 88: 193–7.

McLaughlin K, Jardine AG, Moss JG (2000). ABC of arterial and venous disease. Renal artery stenosis. *British Medical Journal* 320: 1124–7.

CHAPTER 5

CASE 6

INSTRUCTIONS TO CANDIDATES (CASE NOTES)

Name	Peter Hendry
Age	52
Past medical history	Osteoarthritis
	Hypercholesterolaemia
Current medication	Paracetamol 500 mg prn
	Simvastatin 40 mg nocte
Social history	Married, four children

Saw the practice nurse 2 weeks ago for blood pressure and routine blood tests:

Recent blood pressure	137/82 mmHg
Recent blood tests	Hb 14.9 g/dl
	Total cholesterol 3.9 mmol/l
	HDL 1.9 mmol/l
	BMI 30

BRAINSTORM

INSTRUCTIONS TO ROLE PLAYER (PATIENT)

NOT TO BE SEEN BY THE CANDIDATE

You are Peter Hendry, a 52-year-old director of a plumbing firm.

Opening statement:

'Hi Doctor, I'd like to change my cholesterol tablets!'

Patient background:

You are waving a newspaper article.

You have a copy of today's tabloid newspaper.

You highlight an article on statins. The article deems simvastatin an old drug with many side effects.

A new statin, Gold XR, was reviewed in the article. It has been on the market for a week now. A major medical trial, run by the drug company who manufacture Gold XR, concluded that all patients should be switched to the new wonder drug. They claim the drug can reduce deaths from heart disease, stroke, and Alzheimer's disease by 50%.

You are surprised the doctor hasn't heard of the drug.

You would like to have the new statin rather than simvastatin.

You think if the government can pay for polyclinics, there must be millions of pounds in the pot.

You feel you are entitled to the best possible treatment on the NHS as you have paid your taxes.

You don't realise some patients have had to pay for their own chemotherapy; such is the state of the NHS.

You have no idea that the government is squeezing the NHS so much that patients are being refused surgery, eg for varicose veins and hernias.

You hadn't considered that, if the study is sponsored by the drug company, there may be a biased slant to the story.

You are embarrassed as you didn't even think that the newspaper would sensationalise a major health topic.

CHAPTER 5

> *You think 50% improvement is a massive improvement.*
>
> *You don't particularly look after your diet and you don't exercise.*
>
> You say you smoke a little, when asked you admit to *smoking 25 cigarettes a day; you enjoy smoking.*
>
> *You take statins so you don't have to exercise so much and can continue your current unhealthy lifestyle.*

NOTES

DATA-GATHERING, TECHNICAL AND ASSESSMENT SKILLS

- Consider why he requires statins in the first place; in this case it is likely to be a substitute for not exercising and having a poor diet.

- Why does he want to have Gold XL in particular?

- What are his views on his recent cholesterol results? Does he know what they mean?

- What are his views on his lifestyle? Does he think he should change?

- How does he feel about smoking?

- Find out if he knows the about the dangers of smoking (to try and change his view from pre-contemplation to contemplation).

- What are his views on the press and how and why it delivers stories?

- A discussion about what 50% reduction in heart disease, stroke and Alzheimer's disease actually means should take place, first by asking him what he thinks this actually means (eg relative risk reduction).

CLINICAL MANAGEMENT SKILLS

- Consider evaluating his cardiovascular risk and discuss lifestyle changes as an option rather than taking drugs. Be explicit and suggest, if he doesn't mind, that you will talk about the drug later during the consultation (signposting); that way he will feel you are taking his wishes into account.

- Consider referring him to the smoking cessation clinic if he so wishes.

- Advise on weight management or consider referring him to an obesity clinic (see NICE guidelines on obesity).

- It would be reasonable to check a fasting glucose.

- Check MIMS/BNF on Gold XL in front of him, discussing that the drug hasn't reached the national drug formularies.

- Continue simvastatin for the moment.

- It would be inappropriate to change his drug to Gold XL without being satisfied it is clinically indicated, safe, superior in effect to simvastatin, and cost effective.

- You are not obliged to prescribe a drug if you don't think it is appropriate.

- Offer to look at the original research papers on Gold XL and seek advice from the prescribing department at the Primary Care Trust (PCT).

- Once you are more informed about Gold XL, you can drop him a line or invite him in to discuss the matter further. Let him know you will do this if he wishes.

INTERPERSONAL SKILLS

- What are his ideas on why patients are prescribed statins? Is he concerned he may be at risk of cardiovascular disease and therefore wants a statin? If so, why? Does he know what the risk factors are for developing heart disease?

- This isn't an easy consultation and it could easily deteriorate to a conflict unless managed carefully.

- Care should be taken not to be patronising or judgemental. Look out for cues; does he appear angry? If so, acknowledge it, or perhaps change the focus of the discussion back to his agenda.

- Offering choices about lifestyle changes is appropriate. Sharing and agreeing a plan that is suitable to both him and you will enhance his satisfaction in your care. He will need support in changing his lifestyle.

- How would he like to be followed up?

- He may not want to engage in a healthy lifestyle, but continue to take statins.

- Would it be reasonable to prescribe a drug as a mandate for him to continue his current lifestyle? It would seem unethical to deny him his current statin if he doesn't want to change his lifestyle.

Note: Gold XL is a fictitious drug in this case.

CHAPTER 5

PREVENTION OF CARDIOVASCULAR DISEASE JOINT BRITISH SOCIETIES' GUIDELINES

TARGET GROUPS	• Established atherosclerotic CVD • Diabetes • Diastolic BP ≥100 mmHg • TC:HDL ≥6.0	• 10 year CVD risk ≥20% • Systolic BP ≥160 mmHg • Elevated BP + target organ damage • Familiar dyslipidaemia. Specialist care required
ASSESSMENT	• Estimate CVD risk using JBS prediction charts (www.bhsoc.org) • Opportunistic risk assessment in over 40s regardless of history – CVD risk <20% repear within 5 years • CVD risk assessment in younger adults if family history of premature CVD (men <55 years, women <65 years)	

	• Risk assessment should include
	  – Ethnicity
	  – Family CVD history
	  – BP
		– Non-fasting plasma glucose
		– Smoking history
		– Weight and waist circumference
		– Non-fasting lipids of full fasting lipid profile

AIMS	• Reduce BP to <130/80 mmHg in atherosclerotic CVD, diabetes or chronic renal failure • Reduce BP to <140/85 mmHg if asymptomatic and 10-year CVD risk ≥20% • Reduce TC to <4.0 mmol/L or by 25%, whichever is lower • Reduce LDL-C to <2.0 mmol/L or by 30%, whichever is lower • Maintain BMI <25 kg/m² • Maintain waist circumference men <102cm, women <88cm (white Caucasian) • Maintain waist circumference men <90cm, women <80cm (Asian) • Maintain fasting plasma glucose ≤6.0 mmol/L in all high risk patients + HbA1c <6.5% in diabetes	
LIFESTYLE CHANGES	• Lose weight if BMI >25 kg/m² or waist greater than desired limits (see above) • Reduce total fat (≤30% of energy intake); saturated fats (≤10% total fat); increase oily fish consumption • Limit cholesterol to <300mg per day • 5 portions of fruit and vegetables per day • Limit weekly alcohol to ≤21 units (men); ≤14 units (women) • Reduce salt intake to <6.0 g/day • Take regular exercise ie 30 mins + aerobic activity per day most days • Stop smoking	

TREATMENT	• Implement statin therapy to achieve TC and LDL-C targets in patients with:
	  – Atherosclerotic CVD
	  – CVD risk ≥20% but asymptomatic
	  – Diabetes ≥40 years
	  – Diabetes 18–39 years + ≥1 of the following: retinopathy; nephropathy; HbA1c >9%; hypertension; TC ≥6 mmol/L; features of metabolic syndrome; family history of premature CVD
	• Implement aspirin 75mg daily (clopidogrel 75mg daily is aspirin not tolerated) in patients with:
	  – Atherosclerotic CVD (once BP controlled)
	  – CVD risk ≥20% but asymptomatic
	  – Diabetes
	• Ensure glycaemic control in diabetes
	• Treat elevated BP
	• Consider anticoagulants in atherosclerotic CVD + high system embolism risk
	• Implement beta-blocker therapy following MI
	• Implement ACE inhibitor therapy (or antiotensin II antagonish) in heart failure or left ventricular dysfunction
	  – Also in coronary disease and normal LV function if BP not at target
	  – Also in diabetes with renal dysfunction and mictoalbuminuria	

Adapted from JBS2: Joint British Societies guidelines on prevention of cardiovascular disease in clinical practice, 2005.

Fig. 9 Prevention of cardiovascular disease: joint British societies' guidelines. Reproduced with the kind permission of MIMS

CHAPTER 5

LIPID MODIFICATION FOR THE PREVENTION OF CARDIOVASCULAR DISEASE NICE GUIDELINE

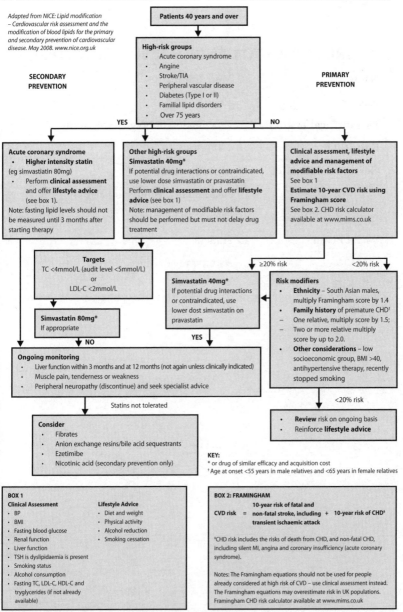

Fig. 10 Lipid modification for the prevention of cardiovascular disease: NICE guidelines. Reproduced with the kind permission of MIMS

CHAPTER 5

CASE 7

INSTRUCTIONS TO CANDIDATES (CASE NOTES)

Name	Meredith Jones
Age	19
Past medical history	Termination of pregnancy, asthma
Best PEFR	420 L/min
Current medication	Microgynon 30°
	Salbutamol CFC-free inhaler
	Clenil Modulite 50°
Social history	Student
	Asthma review due

BRAINSTORM

INSTRUCTIONS TO ROLE PLAYER (PATIENT)

NOT TO BE SEEN BY CANDIDATE

Opening statement:

'Hiya Doc, I think I need some antibiotics.'

Patient background:

You are Meredith Jones, aged 19. You are a law student, in Brighton.

You have had a sore throat for 3 days, prior to which you were well

You have tried many over-the-counter products.

You feel unwell and are getting worse.

You are able to swallow fluids and food.

The infection hasn't affected your asthma and your cough is dry and non-productive.

If at all possible, you would like to avoid taking antibiotics as they always give you thrush. You are happy to take a just-in-case prescription in case it gets really bad.

You are allergic to penicillin – it gives you a rash.

You really came to check it wasn't glandular fever as your best friend died of that after being kicked and his spleen ruptured.

You are not aware antibiotics will render the contraceptive pill less effective.

You take your pill regularly and never miss one.

You say your asthma doesn't bother you.

If asked in more detail, you avoid walking to college but get the bus because you start to wheeze. Come to think of it, you also exercise less because of breathlessness.

Your asthma doesn't affect your sleep.

You don't take your Clenil® regularly and you're not sure what it is for.

You don't use your spacer device and are not sure why it is important.

You have a peak flow meter at home, but you're not sure where it is.

You don't smoke.

NOTES

DATA-GATHERING, TECHNICAL AND ASSESSMENT SKILLS

- It is important to ascertain whether this patient is unwell, and the examination may well offer relevant clinical findings.

- She has symptoms of an upper respiratory tract infection (URTI) but it is important to consider whether she has lower respiratory tract symptoms and signs, particularly given she is asthmatic (auscultate her lungs).

- Severe URTI may present with stridor and/or sepsis. Examination of the throat, assessment for lymphadenopathy and an assessment of systemic involvement should be undertaken; at the very least a temperature and pulse.

- She should be questioned on any drug allergies.

- The latest NICE guidelines on management of upper respiratory tract infections (URTI) is summarised at the end of this section.

- Her clinical record has an overdue asthma review and you should aim to discuss her asthma, if you have time. If you run out of time, it would be good practice to invite her back to see yourself or the practice nurse for a formal asthma review. Much chronic disease follow-up is performed by practice nurses, many of whom will have training in their chosen fields.

- The May 2008 SIGN/British Thoracic Society guidelines on asthma quote the three Royal College of Physicians' questions on asthma control. In the last week (or month):

  - Has your asthma affected your sleep?

  - Have you had your usual asthma symptoms during the day (cough/wheeze/SOB/chest tightness)?

  - Has your asthma interfered with your usual daily activities?

CHAPTER 5

99

Tip

✓ Simply asking: 'How is your asthma doing?' is not acceptable and patients may not realise they are altering their lifestyle to accommodate their symptoms.

Asthma reviews in primary care should also include:

- education

- compliance checks

- review of number of exacerbations

- monitoring, eg with spirometry

- inhaler technique

- formulation of personal management plan.

All too often, patients don't understand the role of each inhaler and the benefits of using a spacer device. Patients' understanding should be checked out.

A smoking and occupational history is important with asthma.

Tip

✓ Asthma remains a life threatening condition and it will undoubtedly feature in the examination in one guise or another. Note the new SIGN/BTS asthma guidelines were published in May 2008.

CLINICAL MANAGEMENT SKILLS

- Her sore throat should be managed by negotiation. It is important to establish what her expectations are; after all many people don't actually want antibiotics but attend for other reasons.

- If an antibiotic is prescribed, she should be warned about the interaction with the oral contraceptive pill.

- If you think she may have glandular fever, it would be appropriate to organise a blood test to confirm this and to discuss the risks of splenic rupture in the mean time.

- Education about asthma, its management (including the role of each inhaler), and then formulating a plan tailored to the individual may improve adherence to medication and reduce symptoms.

- Demonstration on inhaler technique may score points if you have time.

- Measuring peak flow will achieve two things in this scenario. Firstly, to demonstrate to the examiner you know when and how to use a peak flow meter. Secondly, the patient can use it to regularly monitor the effect of using inhaled corticosteroids (via a spacer device).

- Initiating a peak flow diary is helpful; this may help her manage her asthma more effectively.

INTERPERSONAL SKILLS

- It is important to consider what the patient's concerns are. It is easy to assume she wants antibiotics. Her concern is whether she has glandular fever.

- If she does have tonsillitis, rather than giving her a prescription for antibiotics, it would be appropriate to give her options, eg over the counter medications, a delayed prescription or a definite course of medication.

- Appropriate safety netting with respect to both asthma and her URTI is required.

- She should be followed up to assess how she is managing with her asthma.

CHAPTER 5

BTS/SIGN GUIDELINES ON ASTHMA (MAY 2008)

DIAGNOSIS (ADULTS)

- > 1 of wheeze/breathlessness/chest tightness/cough

- Worse at night/with exercise/cold air/allergen exposure

- Atopic history

- Consider with otherwise unexplained low PEFR/FEV_1/eosinophilia

- Undertake reversibility testing with spirometry if uncertainty. Use β-agonists or oral steroids, > 400 ml improvement in FEV_1 suggestive of asthma

- Spirometry preferred to peak flow.

MANAGEMENT

- Control defined as:
    - no day/night symptoms
    - no need for rescue medication/no exacerbations
    - no effect on exercise
    - normal lung function
    - minimal drug side effects.
- Primary prevention:
    - encourage mothers to breast feed
    - avoid tobacco smoke
    - avoid obesity.
- Not enough evidence regarding allergen avoidance, modified milk, vitamins.

CHAPTER 5

- Secondary prevention:
  - reduce house dust-mite
  - allergen specific immunotherapy
  - control of hyperventilation by using the Buteyko breathing – reduces bronchodilator use
  - family therapy.
- Not enough evidence for removing pets/acupuncture/homeopathy/exercise.
- Ionisers have not been shown to be useful.

PHARMACOLOGICAL TREATMENT

- Achieve early control by starting treatment at the appropriate step and then by stepping down to use minimal drugs required to maintain control This is shown in the stepwise approach to asthma management in adults:

Step 1. inhaled β-agonists.

Step 2. add in inhaled corticosteroids (ICS).

Step 3. add in long acting β-agonists (LABA), stop if no effect, increase dose of ICS if effect not adequate – may require leukotriene antagonists or slow release theophylline.

Step 4. increase ICS, add in leukotriene antagonists or slow-release theophylline.

Step 5. oral steroids; refer.

- Ensure compliance and inhaler technique.
- Patients should use the minimal dose of ICS required.
- Consider 'smart' therapy: patients on step 3 who are not well controlled may use budesonide/formoterol rather than short acting β-agonist as rescue, as well as a regular preventative inhaler.
- Short acting β-agonists may be taken prior to exercise.

CHAPTER 5

- Form a management plan with each patient.

- Inhalers and steroids can be used pregnancy.

THE SALMETEROL MULTICENTRE ASTHMA RESEARCH TRIAL (SMART STUDY) 2006

Key points

1. Salmetarol vs placebo

2. Randomised control trial (RCT), 26000 patients

3. Stopped early as increased severe and life threatening exacerbations with salmetarol especially in Afro-Americans

4. ICS seem to be partially protective against this effect. LABAs should not be used without ICS.

NICE GUIDELINES ON RESPIRATORY INFECTIONS, JULY 2008

Key points

1. Manage patients' expectations

2. Offer no prescription, delayed prescription or immediate prescription

3. No/delayed prescription considered for:

    - acute otitis media

    - sore throat

    - tonsillitis

    - common cold

    - sinusitis

- bronchitis.

- reassure antibiotics make little immediate difference and have side effects

- safety net appropriately.

4. Immediate antibiotics may be required depending on clinical presentation in:

- bilateral acute otitis media in children under two

- acute otitis media with discharge

- acute sore throat with three or more Centor criteria:

    - tonsillar exudate

    - tender/inflamed anterior cervical nodes

    - fever

    - absence of cough

- if systemically very unwell

- if complications, eg pneumonia, quinsy, mastoiditis

- if significant co-morbidities:

    - lung/renal/heart disease, eg. heart failure, cystic fibrosis

    - immunosuppressed, ex-premature babies

- > 65 years of age and two of the following or > 80 years of age and one of the following:

    - hospitalised in last year

    - diabetes

    - congestive cardiac failure (CCF)

    - taking steroids.

CHAPTER 5

CASE 8

INSTRUCTIONS TO CANDIDATES (CASE NOTES)

Name   Lucy Ford

Age   29

Medication   Nil

Social history   Social Worker

Last consultation: 6 months ago:

URTI

Paracetamol and steam inhalation advised.

Thinking about getting pregnant, discussed.

BRAINSTORM

INSTRUCTIONS TO ROLE PLAYER (PATIENT)

NOT TO BE SEEN BY THE CANDIDATE

Opening statement:

'I think I may be pregnant doctor, I'm really excited!'

Patient background:

You are Lucy Ford, 29 years old and work as a social worker.

You live with your partner and have been trying for a baby for several months.

You are happy and enjoy your job although it can be challenging.

You are very excited as you have missed a period.

Your last period was exactly 7 weeks ago today.

You have been taking folic acid.

You have stopped smoking.

You have done two pregnancy tests which have been positive, but you would like a confirmatory test by the doctor. Your tests were from the local supermarket and you are convinced they are unreliable.

You have never heard of a pregnancy pack/handheld notes.

You have heard the next step is that you meet the midwife to 'book' the pregnancy.

You don't know you need to avoid soft cheeses and NSAIDS.

You don't know how much alcohol you can drink; you haven't had a drink for 3 months

You have heard of a special scan to check for Down's syndrome but you don't know what it is called. *You would want a termination if it was positive.*

You have had the rubella vaccination at school.

You have never been pregnant before.

You are normally well and have never required gynaecological surgery.

You want to know if you can still go jogging.

You would like to listen to the baby's heartbeat today.

CHAPTER 5

NOTES

DATA-GATHERING, TECHNICAL AND ASSESSMENT SKILLS

- Two pregnancy tests are enough to confirm pregnancy. Another is not required, and you should inform her that the tests in the practice are no more sensitive than the commercially available kits.

- When was her last period?

- Is she taking folic acid, does she know why this is important (education is empowering and can increase compliance)?

- Is she avoiding soft cheese? Does she know why she has to (listeria)?

- Does she know to avoid NSAIDS and why?

- Is she smoking?

- Does she drink alcohol? She should avoid it if at all possible. *The International Journal of Epidemiology* (Oct 2008) recently published data suggesting that, at age 3, children of mothers who drank 1–2 units per week did not exhibit behavioural problems or cognitive deficit and in fact boys had less hyperactivitiy and conduct problems.

- Has she had any abdominal pain or vaginal discharge?

- You may elect to check her blood pressure but it is more common practice to leave to the midwife when she 'books' the pregnancy.

- Has she had any terminations or miscarriages?

- Has she a history of disease that may affect the pregnancy? Cardiac, thyroid, diabetes or pelvic injury?

Tip

✓ You can not always rely on the case summary being complete, as in real life!

CLINICAL MANAGEMENT SKILLS

- Use an obstetric calendar. You can then give her an expected date of delivery.

  Tip

  ✓ **Remember to bring a calendar to the CSA and know how to use it!**

- Discuss that nuchal scans, in addition to blood tests, provide a risk score for Down's syndrome rather than definite yes/no answer.

- She will require a pregnancy pack. (Local practices differ, sometimes doctors give a pack to the woman, and sometimes it is given by the midwife at booking. I suggest you do as you are used to doing.)

- Discuss the process of booking with the midwife and stress that she will need regular appointments with the midwife and doctor over the course of her pregnancy.

- An easy way to confirm pregnancy in the clinic is to 'listen' for a fetal heart beat with a Doppler ultrasound probe. It is too early to detect a heartbeat at 7 weeks unless a vaginal probe is used. A vaginal probe can detect a heartbeat at 5 weeks and 4 days.

- Jogging shouldn't present any problems.

INTERPERSONAL SKILLS

- As in many cases, summarising what you have said, eg the do's and don'ts of pregnancy can help her understanding and reinforce your point. You may want to check her understanding by asking explicitly. As in all consultations, ensure you have understood the patient and the patient has understood you.

- She may or may not take in all of what you say due to the excitement of knowing she is pregnant. Can you offer her any leaflets, websites or an opportunity to come back if she has questions?

- Women are often full of worry during pregnancy. Ample opportunity should be given for her to express her concerns. Some women may be too shy to ask questions outright but instead offer a cue. Be vigilant for cues and actively listen.

- Explaining the sensitivity of pregnancy tests should be done in language she understands.

NICE GUIDELINES ON ANTENATAL CARE, MARCH 2008

KEY POINTS

1. Woman-centred care.

2. Appropriate access to care.

3. Consider 10 mcg vitamin D/day during pregnancy, and during breastfeeding in at risk groups, eg South Asians.

4. All pregnant women should be screened for haemoglobinopathies by 10 weeks into pregnancy.

5. Nuchal scan, human chorionic gonadotropin (hCG) and plasma protein A – for Down's syndrome – should be offered from 11^{+0} to 13^{+6} weeks into pregnancy. If women book later, offer a triple/quadruple test at 15–20 weeks.

6. Consider screening for gestational diabetes in high risk patients, eg high BMI, previous gestational diabetes, family history, previous macrosomic baby, ethnic risk.

7. Those with co-morbidities or previous obstetric complications may require additional care.

8. Advise on alcohol/drugs/smoking.

9. Avoid alcohol for the first 12 weeks of pregnancy if possible.

CHAPTER 5

10. If a woman wants to drink alcohol, the latest NICE guidelines suggest a maximum of 1–2units/week. Avoid binge drinking. However, see page 109 for information on a recently published survey.

11. Offer nicotine replacement therapy.

12. Investigate/treat Hb < 11 g/dl.

13. Not routine:

- breast/pelvic examination
- weighing
- screening for chlamydia/streptococcus B
- fetal movement counting.

CASE 9

INSTRUCTIONS TO CANDIDATES (CASE NOTES)

Name	Barry Kirk
Age	57
Past medical history	Osteoarthritis
	Hypothyroidism
Current medication	Cocodamol 8/500 prn
	Levothyroxine 200 mcg od
Social history	Married, two children

Last thyroid function test:

Two years ago; euthyroid. Reminder letter sent to have blood repeated.

BRAINSTORM

INSTRUCTIONS TO ROLE PLAYER (PATIENT)

NOT TO BE SEEN BY THE CANDIDATE

Opening statement:

'I'd like a PSA test Doctor!'

Patient background:

You are Barry Kirk, aged 57, a company director.

You have wear and tear arthritis which predominantly affects your knees, probably due to years of rugby.

You take cocodamol intermittently for this.

You've had an under active thyroid for many years and take levothyroxine daily for this.

Your weight is stable, you are not sensitive to the heat or the cold and your bowels are normal. Your last thyroid blood test was 2 years ago. You know you ought to have regular tests and you did receive a letter asking you to have one.

You would like a prostate-specific antigen test (PSA).

Your older brother, aged 63, has just been diagnosed with prostate cancer and is scheduled for an operation.

You are worried you may have prostate cancer.

Your brother saw his GP with a poor urinary stream. His PSA was found to be raised. You don't have any more information than that.

Your urinary stream is strong and you don't dribble urine.

You occasionally have to get up in the night to pass urine.

You don't have to wait a while before voiding starts.

You have not lost weight.

You don't suffer from erectile dysfunction.

You don't suffer from any back pain.

As far as you're concerned, a normal PSA excludes prostate and a

> *raised PSA confirms the diagnosis.*
>
> *You take on board what the doctor says about the PSA test, but would still like it done.*
>
> *You don't want a rectal examination if asked.*

NOTES

DATA-GATHERING, TECHNICAL AND ASSESSMENT SKILLS

- The primary focus of this case revolves around the patient's fear of having prostate cancer. As such, to gather some information about his bother's case will help you relate this to his own fears and symptoms. For example, his brother had a poor urine flow. You may want to ask if he has that too.

- A full urological history should be taken. In particular, ask about quality of urine flow, frequency, nocturia, haematuria, hesitancy, terminal dribbling and perineal pain. You should also enquire about back and bone pain, weight loss and erectile dysfunction.

- You may want to explain why you are asking about back pain or else he may not understand your questioning, even though you think you're doing a good job.

- A per rectal examination (PR) would not be allowed in the CSA examination. In any case, disturbing the prostate may elevate the PSA.

- His thyroid functions (TFT) have not been checked in 2 years. You should enquire about why he hasn't had a blood test; was it the failure of the practice to recall him (assuming there is a recall system) or did he omit to have the test? In this case, a letter was sent, did he receive it?

- A cursory review of thyroid symptoms should be taken.

- If appropriate, a brief examination to ensure he is clinically euthyroid would be appropriate, eg check his pulse rate and rhythm. You would not be expected to perform a formal and full thyroid examination in this situation.

Tip

✓ Explain to the patient that you are examining him in order to check if he if he has too much or too little levothyroxine replacement. This will serve to 'sign-post' to the patient what you are doing. Also, it will alert the examiner to what you are doing (like a driving test) and that you are thinking widely.

CLINICAL MANAGEMENT SKILLS

- Explaining the issues around PSA testing is essential, including the concepts of false-negative and false-positive, in a way that the patient understands.

- Reiterating the value of annual TFTs should be reinforced. Does he know why this is required?

- Check PSA (if patient would still like this after your discussion) and TFTs. If he had symptoms such as polyuria or nocturia, a blood glucose would also be reasonable. Hypercalcaemia can also cause polyuria.

- Dip-stick the urine for blood, or at least ask for the nurse to do this when he has his blood test (this will save you time during the examination but more importantly, it is often what we do in daily practice if appropriate).

CHAPTER 5

INTERPERSONAL SKILLS

- The main issue in this case is a discussion about the values of the PSA test. So often patients assume tests have 100% positive and negative predictive values. To convey this in a way the patient understands is clearly very important. To score highly, it is worth checking that the patient understands the issues you have raised regarding PSA.

- Once patients understand that the PSA may be normal in the presence of prostate cancer (up to 20% of cases), and a raised PSA may reflect benign disease but require invasive testing (transrectal biopsy), some may decline the blood test.

- The idea of counselling with respect to the PSA is not necessarily to dissuade patients from having the test, but to inform them of its interpretation.

- This patient is fearful of having cancer. It is important to relieve him of his anxiety or else he will continue to be burdened by fear. He may be reassured by a normal PSA as well as a PR examination. Many patients, despite PSA counselling, will decline a PR on the basis of a normal PSA.

- If his PSA is normal, good safety-netting is required. He should be advised to seek advice if he develops lower urinary tact symptoms or haematuria.

- Check he understands what you mean.

- Appropriate follow-up is required; to discuss the PSA and the thyroid function tests.

CASE 10

INSTRUCTIONS TO CANDIDATES (CASE NOTES)

Name	Sarah Reynolds
Age	39
Past medical history	Coeliac disease
Current medication	Nil
Social history	Non-smoker

BRAINSTORM

INSTRUCTIONS TO ROLE PLAYER (PATIENT)

NOT TO BE SEEN BY THE CANDIDATE

Opening statement:

'I've been getting headaches Doctor.'

Patient background:

You are Sarah Reynolds, a marketing executive.

You're 39, about to have your 40th birthday.

You live on your own and have a very high powered job.

You have had coeliac disease for 20 years and are meticulous about your diet.

You are regularly followed up by your private gastroenterologist and have no complications related to coeliac disease. You don't want to discuss coeliac disease today.

Your headaches have been occurring for 3 months and are getting worse.

They feel like a tight band around your forehead.

The headaches occur almost every day.

They seemed to go while you were away on holiday.

They don't wake you up, but you often find you have them in the mornings.

You don't vomit with them but sometimes feel quite sick.

They do not occur in clusters (clusters = every day for a few days followed by weeks or months without a headache).

You don't suffer any visual disturbance, aura or neurological disturbance.

You do have any neck stiffness.

You don't have a cold.

You haven't been involved in any trauma.

You haven't had your eyes tested in 2 years.

You think you have migraines.

You don't smoke but drink three gin and tonics (1 unit each) to relax at night.

Your last period was 3 weeks ago. They are regular.

You're not sexually active; work is so busy and stressful you don't have time for a relationship. This is upsetting because you're nearly 40 and are desperate to have children. You feel your biological clock is ticking.

You are happy in yourself but work is very stressful. It involves a lot of deadlines and millions of pounds rest on your shoulders.

You find it difficult getting off to sleep, and wake early thinking about work.

You have used your mother's codeine tablets daily to help with the headaches.

NOTES

DATA-GATHERING, TECHNICAL AND ASSESSMENT SKILLS

- The differential diagnosis of headache is vast. In this case the patient has stress headaches.

- The diagnosis is usually made from careful history taking.

- Exclusion of sinister and important conditions is imperative.

- The aetiology of a chronic headache should be borne in mind during the consultation: tension, medication overuse, chronic sinusitis, eye strain/disease, carbon monoxide poisoning, migraine, cluster headaches, raised intracranial pressure (eg neoplastic disease).

- Examination includes blood pressure, fundoscopy, visual fields, head and neck. Examination in her case is normal.

- Her blood pressure should be checked.

- Exclude depression. It is important to ensure she isn't depressed, perhaps by appropriate questioning of biological and cognitive features of depression or by asking her to fill in a validated questionnaire.

- While a short review of her coeliac disease would be appropriate, she is not keen in this case.

Tip

✓ **If this patient was older, temporal arteritis would need to be excluded.**

CLINICAL MANAGEMENT SKILLS

- This patient is likely to have tension headaches secondary to her stressful job. The headaches may also be related to regular analgesia use or eye strain, particularly if she has a busy job and spends hours in front of a computer screen.

- She should be advised to see her optician for an eye check and to refrain from using regular analgesia.

- Her stress should be managed in a way that is suitable to both you and herself. Options include changing her work pattern and counselling.

- Exercise is frequently therapeutic.

- Alcohol can cause headaches, her intake should be discussed.

- You may elect to check her calcium. Hypercalcaemia can cause headache.

CHAPTER 5

INTERPERSONAL SKILLS

- It is crucial to reassure the patient and help her see what the causes of her headaches are likely to be. Many patients with headaches fear a tumour. Her fears should be explored, without assuming what her particular concerns actually are. It would be a catastrophe to make her worried about a condition she hadn't considered. In this case she is concerned about migraine rather than a brain tumour. Migraine should be discussed to put her fears at rest.

- She must feel enabled to choose a management plan that she is comfortable with. By giving her treatment options, she can decide what treatment she prefers.

- Follow-up is essential to check if the headaches have settled and to offer support.

KEY POINTS

1. Migraine

    - periodic headache

    - 80% of patients experience their first migraine before the age 30

    - classical: prodrome, eg mood/appetite change followed by visual/sensory aura

    - common: no aura

    - followed by throbbing unilateral headache, nausea, photophobia, phonophobia

    - lasts 4–72 hours

    - may have unilateral lacrimation

    - reversible neurological signs, eg hemiplegia

    - may result in stroke (rare)

- patient should not have the oral contraceptive pill if patient is at risk of stroke, migraine lasts > 72 hours, focal aura, and those needing ergotamine

- treatment: over-the-counter medication, anti-emetics, $5HT_1$ agonists, and ergotamine.

2. Cluster headaches

- males > females

- onset 25–50 yrs

- clusters last days to weeks, headaches occur daily during this period

- remissions last months

- unilateral severe headache – lasts up to an hour at a time.

- lacrimation and ipsilateral red eye.

- may cause: Horner's syndrome, retro-orbital pain, nasal congestion

- treatment: oxygen, $5HT_1$ agonists,and ergotamine.

- steroids may be used

- verapamil may be used as prophylaxis.

CASE 11

INSTRUCTIONS TO CANDIDATES (CASE NOTES)

Name   Nora Howell

Age   73

Past medical history   Polymyalgia rheumatica, 12 months

Osteoarthritis

Anxiety

Hypertension

Basal cell carcinoma, 2004

Current medication   Prednisolone 8 mg od

Paracetamol 1g qds

Lercanidipine 10 mg od

Social history   Lives by herself

Blood pressure (last week):   138/81 mmHg

Fasting blood sugar (last week):   5.8 mmol/l

Previous consultation:

Malignancy excluded

Normal u/e

Wedge fracture seen on spinal X-ray (T4)

Plan DEXA scan and review

DEXA scan (2 weeks ago): Spinal T score: 2.9

Hip T score: -3.2

Suggest Vitamin D/calcium and bisphosphonates

BRAINSTORM

Tip

✓ If you don't know what the medications are for in the case notes, use your BNF before the patient comes into the room.

INSTRUCTIONS TO ROLE PLAYER (PATIENT)

NOT TO BE SEEN BY THE CANDIDATE

Opening statement:

'Hello Doctor, we've not met before! I've come to get the results of my scan.'

Patient background:

You are Nora Howell, you are 73 years old.

You are a retired dinner lady and live on your own.

Your two children live about 100 miles away.

You have come to get the results of your osteoporosis (DEXA) scan which you had 2 weeks ago.

You've been on prednisolone for a year for polymyalgia rheumatica.

You have had severe back pain for the last 2 months. Your GP organised a lot of blood tests which were normal. An X-ray showed a damaged bone in the back. A scan was organised to look at your bones but you're not exactly sure what it was looking for.

You have not had any weight loss or night sweats.

Your friend has been prescribed prednisolone for a skin disease and she is also taking tablets to help her bones, although you don't know what the tablets do to bones. You are cross that you weren't given bone tablets.

You are currently taking prednisolone (8 mg) every day, although you occasionally forget to take them.

You don't have any muscle stiffness around your neck and shoulders and feel the steroids work well.

You are worried about the bone scan; you were told by one of your friends this was to look for cancer that has spread to the bones, particularly as you had a skin cancer a few years ago.

You have never smoked or drunk alcohol. You have never fallen and are steady on your feet.

NOTES

DATA-GATHERING, TECHNICAL AND ASSESSMENT SKILLS

- The scan results indicate osteoporosis.

- It is likely the patient's osteoporosis has been caused by prednisolone.

- Bisphosphonates ought to have been considered when she was initiated on steroids.

- Other causes of osteoporosis may be considered if relevant:

  - posmenopausal, age-related multiparity, family history, alcohol, smoking, Cushing's, hyperparathyroidism, prolactinoma, hyperthyroidism, ciclosporin, myeloma, ulcerative colitis, renal failure, Tuner's syndrome.

  - DEXA scan compares the patient's bone density to the population mean peak density (eg young adults of same sex).

  - It is expressed as standard deviations (SD) from the mean.

  - T score down to   −1   normal.

  - T score   −1 to −2.5   oesteopenia.

  - T score below   −2.5   osteoporisis.

- Fracture risk increases 2-fold with every SD.

  - Fracture risk increases by 1.5/every 10 years of life over the age of 30.

- Important features to cover include steroid compliance, and ensuring she knows never to stop them suddenly. Does she know why?

- She should be assessed for her risk of falls.

- How is the condition affecting her quality of life?

- Examination of the shoulder girdle and ensuring she doesn't have symptoms of temporal arteritis is appropriate.

CLINICAL MANAGEMENT SKILLS

- Given she has significant osteoporosis with evidence of wedge fracture, calcium and vitamin D supplements in addition to bisphosphonates should be prescribed. The regime (eg weekly alendronate sodium, taken before breakfast while remaining upright) should be explained. Explain the side effects of weekly bisphosphonates and check she is still willing to take them.

- A steroid card should be issued (for the purposes of the examination, you may elect to send one in the post), and it would be prudent to check her understanding of the side effects of steroids.

- An erythrocyte sedimentation rate (ESR) should be organised for polymyalgia rheumatica (PMR) disease monitoring. Her blood pressure and blood glucose should also be monitored regularly.

- If her polymyalgia is quiescent, the prednisolone dose should be reduced to 7 mg od.

- A discussion about pain control (for spinal pain) should take place.

INTERPERSONAL SKILLS

- This patient, perhaps rightly so, is upset that she wasn't given bisphosphonates when she was first commenced on steroids. It would be reasonable to acknowledge her feelings and explore with her what, if anything, she'd like you to do. You may offer to investigate the notes, and it would be good clinical governance to hold a significant event analysis. She may want to hear the outcome of the analysis. This approach is more appropriate than a defensive one.

- She may not fully understand what osteoporosis is. Patients often become confused between osteoarthritis, -porosis and -malacia. Checking out her knowledge of osteoporosis will score highly.

- What are her concerns? In this case, cancer? Can you explain why this isn't cancer, in language she understands and using her own health beliefs? You may start by asking her why she thinks she may have cancer affecting her bones. What is her knowledge of basal cell cancer and its potential for spread?

- Explaining what she may expect from osteoporosis drugs is important. Does she expect them to cure her pain? Does she know how long she has to take the drugs for?

- Discuss her options so management can be shared and she feels empowered.

- It is crucial that you summarise the discussion you have with her and check she understands the issues that have been raised.

- She should be followed up to assess how she is getting on with her medication, and a follow-up DEXA scan may be arranged in the longer term to assess the change in T score.

Tip

✓ NICE guidelines on osteoporosis are pending. It is worth reviewing the NICE website periodically for the latest publications.

CHAPTER 5

CASE 12

INSTRUCTIONS TO CANDIDATES (CASE NOTES)

Name   Unknown

The computers have crashed and you have no access to her notes. You have never met this patient before.

BRAINSTORM

INSTRUCTIONS TO ROLE PLAYER (PATIENT)

NOT TO BE SEEN BY THE CANDIDATE

Opening statement:

'I'd like some more diazepam.'

Patient brakground:

You are Holly Gibbs, aged 22. You are unemployed.

You are very defensive because you are often treated like a drug addict.

You would like a month's supply of diazepam, which you pronounce diazepa<u>n</u>.

You have two children, one of 6 years and another of 3 years.

You live in a rough part of town.

You hate living there; it has a reputation for drug and social problems and you worry about its effect on your children.

You've started an A-level course to make a better life for you and your children.

You don't have time for friends and you find it difficult to trust anyone.

You were fostered from the age of nine, following the death of your parents.

You take diazepam, 5 mg 3 times a day, *for anxiety since being raped 4 years ago.*

You get the shakes if you don't take them.

You never take more than you're supposed to and would love to come off them. You have never sold diazepam to anyone else.

You don't pay for prescriptions.

You saw a psychiatrist and a rape counsellor on a fortnightly basis for a year regarding the rape.

You haven't been sleeping and your appetite and weight have dropped over the last 2 months

You feel your concentration is non-existent and that you can't remember a thing.

You haven't enjoyed life for the last 3 months.

Life is worth living, only for the sake of your children otherwise you'd end it.

You would never harm your children.

You don't hear voices and have no paranoid symptoms.

You have never taken illicit drugs.

You don't drink alcohol or smoke.

You are concerned you may be depressed.

You'd rather not have any more tablets, but you found the counselling helpful and are keen to have more sessions.

You don't have any other medical problems

You are not allergic to any medicines.

NOTES

DATA-GATHERING, TECHNICAL AND ASSESSMENT SKILLS

We realise how reliant we are on technology when it fails.

- Establish her history; how much diazepam does she take, what dose, and why she takes it?

- What is her current mental status?

- Is she depressed or anxious? Ask about features of depression and anxiety.

- Consider using a validated questionnaire to quantify the extent of her depression and anxiety.

- Are there features of bipolar disorder?

- Is she suicidal?

- Is she functioning?

- What is her social status?

- Does she take illicit drugs?

- Who is her usual doctor?

- Is she coping with the children?

- What are her views on diazepam use?

Tip

✓ **The Royal College of General Practitioners offers a course in managing drug misuse; while NICE have published information on addiction, including opiate detoxification and psychological interventions.**

CLINICAL MANAGEMENT SKILLS

- As you don't know her, you may be uncomfortable in prescribing a month's supply of diazepam. It would be reasonable, however, to prescribe a small amount and follow her up regularly until you gain each other's trust.

- Consider weaning her off diazepam, if she is ready to. How would you do that?

- Frequent follow-up, if she agrees, would provide a supportive environment for her.

- Organise counselling or antidepressants, or both, depending on what she wants.

INTERPERSONAL SKILLS

- It is very easy to assume this patient is a drug addict in need of diazepam.

- Apologise for having to take the full history again. Explaining that the computers have crashed will go a long way to making her feel at ease, establishing trust, and making her less defensive.

- Sensitivity to her history is crucial to grain trust.

- What are her concerns? She may be worried about coming off diazepam, in particular she may worry about becoming more anxious, and whether she will ever get better.

- What are her expectations? How will she come off the diazepam? What will happen if she starts to withdraw? What will a counsellor do? Is she concerned anti-depressants are addictive?

- Share management by offering options, eg counselling or antidepressants which will empower her to take control of her health.

- She will need frequent follow-up and support.

CASE 13

INSTRUCTIONS TO CANDIDATES (CASE NOTES)

Name	Joseph Stotter
Age	79
Past medical history	Atrial fibrillation
	Transient ischaemic attack
	Hypertension
	COPD
	Osteoarthritis
	Umbilical hernia repair
	Appendicectomy
	Femoral fracture (road traffic accident, 1978)
Current medication:	Warfarin 3 mg od
	Simvastatin 40 mg nocte
	Ramipril 5 mg od
	Amlodipine 5 mg od
	Bisoprolol 1.25 mg od
	Salbutamol CFC free inhaler
	Tiotropium inhaler 18 mg od
	Paracetamol 500 mg 2 qds
	Tramadol 50 mg 2 qds
Social history	Lives with son and his family
	Wife died 12 years ago
	Retired plumber

Mr Stotter saw Dr Rose last week complaining of upper back pain. He arranged some blood and urine tests:

Hb 10.9 g/dl

ESR 99 mm/Hour

PSA 0.5 ng/ml

Calcium: normal

Protein electrophoresis: monoclonal band

Urine: positive for Bence-Jones protein

BRAINSTORM

Tip

✓ The case notes may appear complicated but read through them carefully, it may be, as in this case, that the majority of the information is background rather than directly relevant to today's consultation.

INSTRUCTIONS TO ROLE PLAYER (PATIENT)

NOT TO BE SEEN BY THE CANDIDATE

Opening statement:

'Hello Doctor, I've come to get my results.'

Patient background:

You are Joseph Stotter, age 79

You've come to get your blood test results; the doctor insisted last week that you come in to get the blood results.

You have been suffering upper back pain for a few months.

The pain has been getting worse and for 2 weeks has been waking you up at night time.

You don't have night sweats but you have lost some weight.

You have not suffered any trauma to your back.

The pain is so bad that paracetamol and tramadol are not controlling the pain.

You have tried physiotherapy and seen a chiropractor with no improvement.

Your urine flow has been normal.

You have had a cough for years, due to your COPD.

You have never coughed up any blood.

Your bowels are normal.

You don't want any blood tests; you want a scan for osteoporosis.

Your wife had osteoporosis and you are convinced that is what you have.

You have no idea what the blood tests were for, you think they were for osteoporosis.

You have started smoking again but you never smoke near the grandchildren and only smoke outside.

You never drink alcohol.

NOTES

DATA-GATHERING, TECHNICAL AND ASSESSMENT SKILLS

- This patient has come to the get the results of his blood tests.

- While it is important to review his history, the focus of the consultation is to manage a new diagnosis of myeloma.

- Given he has back pain, how severe is it? What medications is he taking? Does he get side effects? Does he have leg weakness or experience difficulty in passing urine?

CLINICAL MANAGEMENT SKILLS

- This patient has anaemia, a monoclonal band on protein electrophoresis and Bence-Jones proteins in his urine (note: in around 20% of cases, patients will have Bence-Jones proteins without a monoclonal band. It is therefore imperative urine is sent for Bence-Jones protein if myeloma is suspected).

- It would seem reasonable to recheck his Hb to see if there is a downward trend, to recheck calcium (often raised in myeloma), and renal function ('myeloma kidney').

- Analgesia should be discussed.

- A 2WW referral should be made to the haematology department.

INTERPERSONAL SKILLS

- As with every patient, welcome the patient, make them feel at ease.

- Asking the patient the story so far may put him at ease and give him the opportunity to express his concerns (eg osteoporosis). It will also provide an ideal starting point to the consultation. Check his understanding; does he actually know what osteoporosis is?

- Does he look concerned? Does he offer a cue: 'You look worried…is there something on your mind…'

- Part of the consultation is about breaking bad news. It may be more appropriate for you to explain that you think there is 'something worrying…something more sinister than osteoporosis…a lesion in your back' and see what his reaction is.

- You may want to involve his health beliefs, 'the tests show something more serious than osteoporosis.'

- Check his understanding; does he understand your concern that he has a potentially serious illness?

- You may need to be more explicit, but be sensitive…'the hospital will need to confirm it, but I think you may have a type of cancer in your back…'

- Offer hope: 'The diagnosis still needs to be confirmed…there are treatments available.'

- Sensitivity is important.

- The use of silence is useful.

- Does he have concerns? Will he die? What will the treatment be? Will his pain get worse? How long has he got…? This consultation can easily run over 10 minutes: time management is important. It would be worth explaining that the diagnosis has to be confirmed first and these are questions which the specialist is better placed to answer.

CHAPTER 5

- Would he like to come back soon, perhaps with a family member and for a longer appointment, to discuss the matter further?

- Is he agreeable to an urgent referral?

- What are his expectations? Does he know/want to know what the hospital process is? He may need a marrow biopsy.

- He should contact the surgery if he doesn't hear from the hospital within the week.

- Confirm his contact details so the hospital sends the appointment to the right address.

Chapter 6
Exam Circuit 2

CASE 1

INSTRUCTIONS TO CANDIDATES (CASE NOTES)

You are a locum doctor, you have never met this patient before.

Name	Robin Greeves
Age	39
Past medical history	Recurrent mechanical back pain
	MRI (back) 3 months ago: normal
Current medication	Ibuprofen
Social history	Postman, married, two children

BRAINSTORM

INSTRUCTIONS TO ROLE PLAYER (PATIENT)

NOT TO BE SEEN BY THE CANDIDATE

Opening statement:

'I need a doctor's certificate.'

Patient background:

You are Robin Greeves. You are 39 years old and you work as a postman.

You have suffered from recurrent back pain for the last 8 years since falling off a chair.

You have seen a specialist and been thoroughly investigated, including blood tests and a recent MRI scan.

You have taken many days off work over the years.

Your manager is unhappy about the number of days you have taken off in the past.

You last saw a doctor 3 months ago, for a certificate.

You have come to get another medical certificate.

You want the certificate to cover you for last week, backdated to 7 days ago.

Your pain is better now.

It was the same pain as you always get.

You have no problems passing urine, no numbness or pins and needles.

If you don't get a doctor's certificate, you run the risk of being disciplined or even sacked.

You couldn't come in last week to get a certificate because you were in too much pain and you didn't want to bother the doctor for a home visit. You took paracetamol for the pain.

NOTES

DATA-GATHERING, TECHNICAL AND ASSESSMENT SKILLS

- The patient hasn't come to discuss back pain but to get a medical certificate.

- A Med 5 may be given had he seen a doctor in the last month, and if the notes warrant a certificate.

- How does he manage his pain?

- Ask why he didn't seek advice when he was in pain; that's what most people do.

- Is he aware of the rules surrounding medical certification? Does he know about the rules on self certification?

- Is he aware that doctors may be investigated if they issue certificates fraudulently?

CLINICAL MANAGEMENT SKILLS

- A medical certificate cannot be given on the basis of a patient's own say so.

- A Med 3 certificate cannot be given retrospectively. Many patients don't appreciate this.

- He may be given a private letter stating he was unwell with back pain the previous week. GPs may charge for this.

INTERPERSONAL SKILLS

- This can be a challenging consultation: testing a doctor's probity and knowledge of medical certification.

- It would be easy to give the patient a certificate but that would not be in keeping with the rules stated in the obligations for doctors to issue certificates (see document IB204, available online)

- Knowingly issuing a certificate would be inappropriate irrespective of the consequences for the patient. Telling him you are obliged to operate by the rules (set out in IB204), and that not doing so may lead to sanctions being brought against you, is likely to pacify him.

- It may be helpful to educate the patient on rules surrounding medical certificates.

- Offering the option of a private letter stating the patient's story may be acceptable to him.

- If he gets aggressive, when a Med 3 is not given, it is worth acknowledging how frustrating it must be for him.

- However guilty he makes you feel, you should not break the rules set out in the IB204 document.

CHAPTER 6

CASE 2

INSTRUCTIONS TO CANDIDATES (CASE NOTES)

Name	Annette Johnson
Age	35
Past medical history	Ovarian cancer, curative surgery 4 weeks ago.
Social history	Single, solicitor

BRAINSTORM

INSTRUCTIONS TO ROLE PLAYER (PATIENT)

NOT TO BE SEEN BY THE CANDIDATE

Opening statement:

'I'd like to give you something.'

Patient background:

You are Annette Johnson, you are 35 years old. You live alone and have a very busy job as a solicitor.

You appear anxious.

You have come to the doctor to express your gratitude for diagnosing your ovarian cancer. The doctor's prompt action meant you could have curative surgery.

You are so thankful for the care you received.

You have heard of many legal cases where the doctor has failed to diagnose the cancer and you understand it is a notoriously difficult cancer to diagnose early.

You have made a full recovery and have been back at work for a week.

Things are going well at work and you are very happy there. Your boss is being very supportive.

You would like to express your gratitude by giving the doctor a watch – the watch is worth £200.

You won't take no for an answer.

You feel you owe your life to your doctor.

You understand it is against the general medical council (GMC) guidelines but you won't say anything to them.

You are scared the cancer may return.

You have recurrent nightmares about dying and being in pain.

You also have nightmares about never having children, although you have been told you should be able to conceive with help.

You don't feel depressed.

You are eating well.

You sometimes get panic attacks, they come out of the blue, last a few minutes, and you feel you breathless; as if you are going to die.

You are seeing your oncologist next week.

NOTES

DATA-GATHERING, TECHNICAL AND ASSESSMENT SKILLS

* Little knowledge about ovarian cancer is required in this case.

* It would be good practice to ask how she is doing and assess if she has come to terms with her condition.

* Panic attacks are commonplace; it is not surprising she is suffering from them. What brings them on?

* Anxiety and depression often coincide, screening for depression would be appropriate.

* Quantifying how severe her depression and anxiety is by a validated questionnaire is appropriate.

CLINICAL MANAGEMENT SKILLS

* You may want to offer her counselling or SSRIs for her panic attacks.

* Self-help books and websites such as Moodgym (http://moodgym. anu.edu.au/welcome) are invaluable and empowering.

INTERPERSONAL SKILLS

* She should be followed up appropriately regarding her panic attacks.

* Exploring her ideas about how and why people (and herself) get panic attacks may be therapeutic.

- Many patients fear being prescribed psychiatric drugs. Often, when given the choice, patients prefer non-pharmacological management. Sharing management options will empower her.

- Accepting an expensive gift can adversely affect the doctor-patient relationship and may be considered a conflict of interest. There have been a number of GMC cases surrounding this subject. The Social Care Bill (2000) legislated that gifts over £100 in value should be declared.

- A gift may alter the dynamic between the doctor and patient such that the patient may expect preferential treatment and the doctor feels beholden.

- Explaining to the patient that receiving such gifts would not be in keeping with guidance set out by the GMC would be appropriate. While she may insist you take the watch, it would be advisable to stick with the GMC guidance in a way that won't cause offence and maintain your professional integrity.

CHAPTER 6

CASE 3

INSTRUCTIONS TO CANDIDATES (CASE NOTES)

You are a locum in a busy general practice. One of the partners in the practice has a very good reputation in managing musculo-skeletal disorders.

Name	Henry Carter
Age	39
Past medical history	Recurrent ear infections
	Ankle sprain
	Stress at work
	Tibial fracture (road traffic accident 1992)
Social history	CEO, Carter Computers International

BRAINSTORM

INSTRUCTIONS TO ROLE PLAYER (PATIENT)

NOT TO BE SEEN BY THE CANDIDATE

Opening statement:

'I'd like to see a specialist.'

Patient background:

You are Henry Carter, the owner of a successful computer company.

You have had left shoulder pain for the past 4 months.

You are right handed.

The shoulder also feels stiff and you can't move it as much you normally can; even reaching to your back pocket is difficult.

It is starting to affect your quality of life.

It is affecting your sleep, waking you when you turn. You can't lie on your left side.

Your performance at work is suffering.

You are getting short tempered and your girlfriend made you come to the doctor.

You have recently started going to the gym and think your pain may be related to weight training, although you haven't been able to train recently, because of the pain.

You have heard of a frozen shoulder, but you are not quite sure what it is.

You would like a referral to an orthopaedic consultant. You don't have private insurance as you believe in the NHS, although you think the Labour Government has destroyed it.

When the doctor examines your left shoulder it is painful, especially when it is rotated outwards with your elbow held at 90 degrees (external rotation). It is painful whether the doctor moves it or if you move it yourself.

CHAPTER 6

NOTES

DATA-GATHERING, TECHNICAL AND ASSESSMENT SKILLS

- This patient describes an adhesive capsulitis of the shoulder.

- It is relevant to explore how the pain came about and the effect on his quality of life.

- The assessment should include an examination of the shoulder in order to exclude other pathologies and to confirm the diagnosis.

- It is important to inspect the shoulder to ensure there are no scars or swellings. Is there any muscle wasting?

- Is there any evidence of tenderness, crepitus or effusion within the joint and supporting structures?

- Check the patient's range of movements, active and passive. They should be seated comfortably.

- Assess the joints, rotator cuff, and for a frozen shoulder.

- The diagnosis of adhesive capsulitis is a clinical one.

CLINICAL MANAGEMENT SKILLS (ADHESIVE CAPSULITIS)

- Analgesia, paracetamol, NSAIDS.

- TENS machine.

- Physiotherapy if combined with intra-articular injection of steroid.

- Patient education.

INTERPERSONAL SKILLS

- This patient would like to see an orthopaedic surgeon. What does he hope to gain from this?

- Establishing what the patient knows about 'frozen shoulder' and educating him on its pathology and treatment is empowering. Based on this new knowledge, he may change his view about wanting a referral to an orthopaedic surgeon. Offer leaflets to reinforce what you have said.

- What are his expectations? Symptoms may persist for up to 3 years.

- Offering management options before a surgical referral will again empower the patient and make him feel involved in is own care.

- Inviting the patient to see your colleague (which can be organised quickly) who has a special interest in musculo-skeletal diseases and who is used to managing his condition is entirely appropriate.

- If he is still keen to see an orthopaedic surgeon, it may be worth indicating that the surgeon may also try an injection, but it may take several weeks before he is seen.

- Side effects of NSAIDS should be discussed.

DERBY VOCATIONAL TRAINING SCHEME FOR GENERAL PRACTICE

CHAPTER 6

CASE 4: TELEPHONE CONSULTATION

INSTRUCTIONS TO CANDIDATES (CASE NOTES)

Name	Thomas Protheroe
Age	19
Past medical history	Asthma
	Two previous admissions to intensive care for asthma
Current medication	Salbutamol
	Fluticasone propionate and salmeterol combined inhaler
Social history	Student, lives with parents

BRAINSTORM

INSTRUCTIONS TO ROLE PLAYER (PATIENT)

NOT TO BE SEEN BY THE CANDIDATE

Opening statement:

'Hi Doctor, I want a home visit for my son.'

Patient background:

You are Mrs Protheroe, Thomas' mother.

You called the doctor for a home visit (panicking).

He has a sore throat and a fever.

You would like a home visit.

You don't think he is well enough to talk to the doctor himself, his throat is too sore.

You refuse to let the doctor speak to him, despite the doctor's efforts.

He has had a sore throat for 2 days.

He hasn't taken any over the counter drugs, except for lozenges.

He is alert and his breathing is fine.

He isn't wheezing.

He isn't dribbling and has managed to eat some soup.

He hasn't done a peak flow.

If asked to do so, the peak flow is 600 l/min (best is 620 l/min).

He also has a headache.

He doesn't have any neck stiffness or photophobia.

He is alert and his hands aren't cold.

You can't see a rash.

Your thermometer is broken but he feels hot.

He is laid up on the sofa and you don't feel he is well enough to come to the surgery.

You are worried that if he goes out of the house, he may catch a chill and develop a chest infection.

You understand that GPs are busy and you don't like to call the doctor out but, you don't want your son to travel.

You know how much GPs are paid and you feel it's your right to have a visit.

You will complain to the PCT and newspapers if you don't get a visit.

NOTES

DATA-GATHERING, TECHNICAL AND ASSESSMENT SKILLS

- It is difficult to take a history over the phone.

- It is even more difficult when the history is taken from a third party.

- He is hot and despite the unavailability of a thermometer, it is feasible he as a fever.

- He has a sore throat and it is likely he has an upper respiratory infection.

- The fact that Thomas is not dribbling is important, as dribbling could indicate significant upper respiratory disease which may require hospital management.

- He has a headache and evidence of meningism should be explored.

- He should be assessed for symptoms of sepsis.

- He has brittle asthma, one should ensure he is not in respiratory distress.

CLINICAL MANAGEMENT SKILLS

- Over the counter drugs (avoiding NSAIDS as he as brittle asthma) may be advised.

- Assessing him over the phone through a third party is difficult. Failure to visit and failure to examine are common causes for complaints against doctors. If you are unable to assess the patient adequately, and his mother refuses to bring him to the surgery, a home visit should be arranged.

- The GMC advises that a clinician should always justify their actions and adequately assess their patients (www.gmc-uk.org/guidance/good_medical_practice/GMC_GMP.pdf)

INTERPERSONAL SKILLS

- It would be helpful to explore why his mother is reluctant to bring her son to the surgery. Perhaps her ideas can be discussed and her concerns dealt with.

- A home visit may incur a delay in his care if there are other visits to deal with. He could be seen more quickly if she brought him in. By explaining this to her, she may be persuaded to bring him in.

- She has made life difficult by not allowing you to speak to her son. Irrespective of the legalities of consent, given you have not been able to speak to him, you have a duty of care to the patient. If the patient is apparently too unwell to come to the surgery and you can not persuade the mother to bring him in, you have little choice but to see him at home.

- Appropriate safety-netting should be discussed until you arrive at the patient's house.

CASE 5

INSTRUCTIONS TO CANDIDATES (CASE NOTES)

Name	May Connolly
Age	79
Past medical history	Mild COPD
Current medication	Salbutamol prn
	Ipratoprium bromide qds
Social history	Widowed
	FEV$_1$: 70% predicted

BRAINSTORM

INSTRUCTIONS TO ROLE PLAYER (PATIENT):

NOT TO BE SEEN BY THE CANDIDATE

Opening statement:

'I'm so embarrassed Doctor, I've been bleeding from my back passage.'

Patient background:

You are May Connolly, you are 79 years old.

You live on your own.

You have severe lung disease due to smoking for 40 years of your life.

You no longer smoke.

You have been bleeding from you back passage for the last month.

The blood tends to be mixed in with the stool.

You have had more diarrhoea lately, for about 3 months.

You have been experiencing mild abdominal pains in the right side if your 'stomach.'

You pressed on your abdomen yourself and felt a lump there.

Your weight is going down and you've felt tired lately.

You know in your heart you have cancer, but know little about the condition.

You want it confirmed so you can organise your Will.

You would like to be referred to hospital for investigations, but you are worried about having surgery or chemotherapy.

Will these treatments be painful? Will you lose your hair and get infections? You know someone who had chemotherapy and they suffered with infections and ulcers in their mouth.

You aren't depressed or suicidal.

You have had a good life and you are not afraid to join your husband, who died last year.

You don't want to have any intimate examinations today.

You can't remember what your parents died from.

NOTES

DATA-GATHERING, TECHNICAL AND ASSESSMENT SKILLS

- This patient has red flag symptoms suggestive of bowel malignancy. These should be asked for in detail:

  - rectal bleeding in absence of anal symptoms

  - change in bowel habit especially to looser stool

  - weight loss

  - tenesmus

  - obstruction

  - palpable mass.

- Abdominal examination is essential in this situation, not only to confirm her own findings of a mass (assume she has a malignant feeling mass for the purposes of this case, of course, the role player would not have positive clinical signs), but to assess its characteristics and check for hepatomegaly.

- A brief review of her conjunctivae would be reasonable as a gross sign of anaemia.

- Are there signs of acute bowel obstruction?

- She does not want a rectal examination and her wishes should be respected.

CLINICAL MANAGEMENT SKILLS

- A 2WW cancer referral is appropriate, if she agrees.

- This patient suspects she has cancer. While it is likely, one should offer hope and explain the diagnosis needs to be confirmed.

- Baseline bloods should be organised. In particular, full bloods count. If she is anaemic, she should be commenced on iron supplements (you shouldn't routinely commence iron replacement unless the aetiology of the anaemia is known). If required, Mrs Connolly may be amenable to having a blood transfusion as a day case or perhaps at a local hospice.

- Her pain should be managed appropriately.

- Introduction to community cancer nurses would offer her support (once the diagnosis is confirmed).

- Explain the symptoms of bowel obstruction and what she should do if this arises, eg go to nearest A/E department or contact the practice.

INTERPERSONAL SKILLS

- Agree that she is likely to have cancer, but explain this will still need to be diagnosed in secondary care. What is her knowledge base? Does she know what bowel cancer is and what it means? What would she like to know? This will need to be done sensitively.

- Explore her concerns, in this case about treatment. If her fears of surgery are addressed, she may agree to have active treatment.

- Ensure she is not depressed; she may refuse treatment as she wants to die. This isn't the case with this patient.

- Is she aware of the consequences of not having treatment? Unchecked spread of the condition, risk of bowel obstruction, and death.

- Is she happy to be seen in hospital? Does she know what to expect? Does she know she is not obliged to have any treatment if she doesn't want it?

- She should be made aware she can change her mind about treatment any time.

The GMC has published new guidance – *Consent: patients and doctors making decisions together*[1] which is relevant to many of the cases in general practice.

CHAPTER 6

SUMMARY OF *CONSENT: PATIENTS AND DOCTORS MAKING DECISIONS TOGETHER*

REVIEWED BY DR RAJ THAKKAR, GMC TODAY, MAY 2008

'Patient-centred consulting' dictates we consider our patients' views and value their beliefs. By placing their illness in the context of their life and considering their ideas, concerns and expectations we enhance the patient experience.

The GMC's new guidance focuses on the principles of patient-centred consulting and emphasises working in partnership with patients. It's no surprise that many of the concepts described in the document are familiar to those versed in classic GP consulting models such as the one described in The New Consultation by Pendleton et al.

For some GPs, very little will change. After all, this is how many GPs consult routinely. More time may be needed with every patient to ensure we gauge how much information they would like to know about their illness, take into account their health beliefs and finally inform them of the pros and cons of each treatment modality.

While intuition often tells us how much information a patient would like, patient-centred consulting dictates one should explore this with the patient. Information should then be delivered with clarity, perhaps with the assistance of interpreters, diagrams and leaflets.

We must respect our patients' decisions, refrain from being judgemental and forge trusting professional relationships with them. Assessing capacity in line with the Mental Capacity Act 2005, managing patients who lack capacity and consent of those under the age of 18 are helpfully discussed in the guidance.

In order to make a decision about their treatment, patients need to be adequately informed about the condition itself, risks of not treating and the risks of each treatment. Doctors are therefore required to possess knowledge and hence keep up-to-date.

CHAPTER 6

Equally as important, skills are required to communicate the risks in ways patients understand. While doctors should inform patients of risk, one has to maintain perspective and offer a balanced view. When explaining serious risks, one ought to present the likelihood of the adverse event occurring, what symptoms and signs to be aware of, and management and prognosis of the adverse outcome.

Scaring our patients, however, may only act to confuse and perhaps inadvertently dissuade them from accepting vital treatment. Doctors should, nevertheless, respect their patients' treatment choice, even if it is not in their best medical interest, so long as they are of sound mind.

The GMC's guidance acts to empower patients and deliver a more satisfying service. Doctors are obliged to embrace it, move with the times and provide a robust and first class service

Reproduced with kind permision of the GMC.

CHAPTER 6

CASE 6

INSTRUCTIONS TO CANDIDATES (CASE NOTES)

You are a locum doctor at a busy practice

Name	Sarah Mullen
Address	11 Archway Road
	Marble Hill
Age	37
Past medical history	Nil
Social history	Married

Last entry 6 months ago (practice nurse):

Smear taken

Full sweep

Cervix visualised

Result:

Severe dyskaryosis – normal, no action

BRAINSTORM

INSTRUCTIONS TO ROLE PLAYER (PATIENT)

NOT TO BE SEEN BY THE CANDIDATE

Opening statement:

'Hello Doctor, I'm a little worried, I've been bleeding.'

Patient background:

You are Sarah Mullen and you are 37 years old.

You are a secretary at the local factory.

You live with your husband *and are in a happy and committed relationship.*

You don't have children but you're hoping to try soon.

You have noticed abnormal vaginal bleeding for the last 3 months.

It has been getting worse recently and you have noticed some blood clots.

You have noticed bleeding in between periods and also after sexual intercourse.

Your last smear was 6 months ago. You thought nothing of the bleeding initially as you thought your smear was normal.

You understood the surgery's policy was to contact patients if smears were abnormal.

As the symptoms persisted, you thought you should get checked out.

You would like to double check whether the results of the smear were normal.

When you learn about the abnormal result, you would like to know why you weren't informed.

You want to know how this will affect your fertility and what the cause of the bleeding is likely to be.

You would like to know what the practice is going to do about the situation.

You would rather not have an examination today.

You would like a referral to a gynaecologist: you have private insurance.

NOTES

DATA-GATHERING, TECHNICAL AND ASSESSMENT SKILLS

- A detailed menstrual history is essential.

- Does she have any red flag symptoms suggesting malignancy?

- It is helpful to establish exactly where she had her smear done and by whom.

- Has she moved and has the practice got her right address?

- Was there any evidence in the notes that any action was taken on the abnormal smear result?

CLINICAL MANAGEMENT SKILLS

- This patient shows concerning symptoms.

- She ought to have a full blood count.

- The most important act is to exclude a gynaecological malignancy.

- Organising a quick referral letter to her private consultant is appropriate.

INTERPERSONAL SKILLS

- Her wishes regarding examination should be respected.

- What are her ideas and concerns? Does she have any idea this may represent a malignancy?

- She has private insurance and a referral to a gynaecologist is indicated. Does she have a specialist in mind, or would she like a recommendation? Does she know the process of how to organise a private referral? For example she will have to ring her insurance company to obtain an authorisation code, and also contact the private hospital to organise an appointment.

- It is likely she will be angry and upset.

- Does she have any views on what she would like you to do? She may not want to take the matter further, or she may make a complaint or even bring legal action against the practice.

- It will be difficult as a locum to resolve the situation. Tell the patient you will bring it to the attention of the partners and practice manager. A full investigation (significant event analysis) should be held.

CASE 7

INSTRUCTIONS TO CANDIDATES (CASE NOTES)

You are new to the practice; it is your first day as a salaried doctor.

Name	Perry Smith
Age	61
Past medical history	MI 3 years ago
Current medication	Aspirin 75 mg od
	Ramipril 10 mg od
	Simvastatin 40 mg nocte
	Atenolol 100 mg od
	Tadalafil 10 mg prn
Social history	Married, four children

Last entry in notes:

'Invite patient to come in to discuss meds. He should not have been getting tadalafil on NHS as per practice audit on phosphodiesterase inhibitors. Need to prescribe privately only. Doesn't fulfil 'SLS' criteria"

BRAINSTORM

INSTRUCTIONS TO ROLE PLAYER (PATIENT)

NOT TO BE SEEN BY THE CANDIDATE

Opening statement:

'Hi Doctor, I've not met you before, my old doctor has retired. I've been asked to come in to discuss my tablets.'

Patient background:

You are Perry Smith, you are 61 years old.

You are a carpenter, although business hasn't been good recently.

You have no idea what the issue is regarding your medication.

You are shocked and upset when the doctor says you need to pay for your tadalafil.

You have been taking them since your heart attack.

It transformed your marriage which is brilliant at the moment. Prior to the tablets, your erectile dysfunction was seriously affecting your relationship.

You don't understand why you got them for free up until now.

You are over 60 and think you're entitled to free prescriptions.

You can't afford to pay for them.

If you don't have them it will destroy your marriage and you will get depressed.

You use about 2 tablets a week.

You want to know how this could have happened.

What practice systems are in place to ensure this doesn't happen?

You wonder what do other men do, and how can you get them for free?

You have heard you can buy them over the internet, you wonder what the doctor's views are on this.

You would like the practice to pay some of the prescription as a gesture of good will.

> *You would like to know if there anything else that could help with erectile dysfunction.*
>
> *You don't suffer any chest pain when you exert yourself.*
>
> *You don't have a tremor.*
>
> *You have a good urine flow.*
>
> *You have a good sex drive.*
>
> *Your nipples don't leak fluid.*
>
> *You don't have to get up in the night to pass urine and your weight is stable.*
>
> *You are happy, although you have a few financial pressures.*
>
> *You drink half a bottle of wine per night. No more on weekends.*
>
> *You don't smoke.*
>
> *You don't exercise.*

NOTES

DATA-GATHERING, TECHNICAL AND ASSESSMENT SKILLS

- Establish his use of tadalafil, eg 2 tablets/week.

- Understand his knowledge of the current NHS prescribing guidelines with respect to phosphodiesterase inhibitors for erectile dysfunction.

- Does he have any symptoms suggestive of conditions entitling him to free tadalafil?

- Was he ever checked for causes of erectile dysfunction by his previous GP?

Tip

- ✓ Make use of the BNF in this consultation – it will list those entitled to free tadalafil. These include:

    - ✓ those receiving the drug before 14 February 1998

    - ✓ those suffering from:

        - ✓ diabetes

        - ✓ multiple sclerosis

        - ✓ Parkinson's disease

        - ✓ polio

        - ✓ prostate cancer

        - ✓ severe pelvic injury

        - ✓ single gene neurological disease

        - ✓ spina bifida

        - ✓ spinal cord injury

        - ✓ patients having dialysis or having had a renal transplant for renal failure

        - ✓ previous prostatectomy or radical pelvic surgery.

- Consider other causes of erectile dysfunction in the history.

- How much alcohol does he drink? This may be contributing to his erectile dysfunction? Is he aware if this?

- Is he depressed?

- Does he have symptoms of prostatism, diabetes or thyroid disease?

- Does he have low libido? Does he have galactorrhoea (prolactinoma)?

CHAPTER 6

CLINICAL MANAGEMENT SKILLS

- It may be reasonable to change his atenolol to a cardioselective β-blocker or to reduce his atenolol to a lower dose. This may be the underlying cause of his erectile dysfunction. His pulse and blood pressure should be checked and he should be warned about unmasking angina if his β-blockers are altered.

- Discuss a reduction in alcohol as a form of treatment.

- Exercise should be encouraged, although he should be warned about angina.

- Arranging a series of baseline bloods (FBC, glucose, prolactin, testosterone, TFTs, PSA) and the use of a depression screening tool may appropriate.

INTERPERSONAL SKILLS

- This is a difficult case to manage on your first day.

- You have to break it to him that he has to pay for his drugs. This should be done sensitively.

- Giving him options about improving his erectile dysfunction may give him hope and pacify him eg reducing or changing his atenolol and changing his lifestyle. Other options would be to check him for underlying causes such as diabetes and prostate disease. Once given options, he should feel enabled to choose what suits him.

- It is a mistake by the practice, and admitting this was a regrettable oversight is not unreasonable.

- The practice cannot pay for his drugs.

- Explaining the system to him, and perhaps suggesting he was fortunate to have received free tadalafil up until now, may make him see the positive side of the situation. This could come across in an aggressive tone and you should be careful to say it in a passive tone.

- Explaining that all patients in the practice, who have been inappropriately prescribed tadalafil free on the NHS, have been contacted may make him feel less victimised.

- You may offer to carry out a significant event analysis and write to him with the outcome.

- Appropriate follow-up reviewing the results of your action plan (including to check if he is experiencing angina) is essential.

CASE 8

INSTRUCTIONS TO CANDIDATES (CASE NOTES)

You have never met this patient before.

Name	Elizabeth Ross
Age	49
Past medical history	Depression
Current medication	Citalopram 20 mg od
Social history	Store manager

BRAINSTORM

INSTRUCTIONS TO ROLE PLAYER (PATIENT)

NOT TO BE SEEN BY THE CANDIDATE

Opening statement:

'I've come to get my tablets Doctor.'

Patient background:

You are Elizabeth Ross, you are 49 years old.

You have depression.

You have run out of antidepressant tablets.

You normally get a month's worth at a time.

You have been taking citalopram for 8 months ever since your husband admitted he was having an affair. You are still with him and things between you are slowly improving.

You haven't taken your tablets for 5 days as you think you may be getting side effects. You don't feel you have any withdrawal effects.

You sleep until 7 am, but you find it difficult to get off to sleep.

Your concentration and memory aren't what they should be and you feel its impacting your performance at work.

You are eating well and your weight is stable. Your mood is worse in the mornings.

You and your partner are starting to have a physical relationship again. You haven't been able to reach orgasm and you think that may be due to the tablets, but you are very embarrassed to ask about that.

You feel guilty that you haven't fully forgiven your partner.

He never hits you.

You would like to stay with him and are sure the future is promising; you are just not there yet. You are not suicidal.

You don't think citalopram is right for you; you feel emotionally numbed and would like to have counselling, you have heard counselling is very effective.

You have been drinking more alcohol lately, to help with you sleep. You don't have panic attacks or obsessional thoughts, although you sometimes think about your partner with another woman. You are a little anxious but it's not that bad at the moment.

You haven't been drinking this much for long and you know it's wrong. You feel bad about drinking this much. You drink a 750 ml bottle of 12% wine per night. You think each bottle has 5 units but you are not sure. You only drink in the evenings and never drink and drive. Your partner hasn't commented on your drinking.

NOTES

DATA-GATHERING, TECHNICAL AND ASSESSMENT SKILLS

- It is important to establish the background to her depression and what her current symptoms are. Check for biological (sleep disturbance, diurnal-mood variation, concentration and memory disturbance, loss of libido), cognitive (guilt, poor outlook for the future, low self esteem, anxiety, suicidal ideation), and if appropriate psychotic (auditory hallucinations, delusions) features.

- You may want to use a validated questionnaire, if available, such as the Hospital Anxiety and Depression score (HAD) – recent evidence suggests questionnaires such as this have a very good negative predictive value.

- A suicidal risk assessment is important.

- Does she feel is she improving or getting worse? If not, why not?

- How is she managing with her tablets? Is she taking them regularly? Does she have any side effects?

- Establish how much alcohol she is actually drinking. This can be done using the formula in figure 11.

- How is her situation affecting her quality of life?

CHAPTER 6

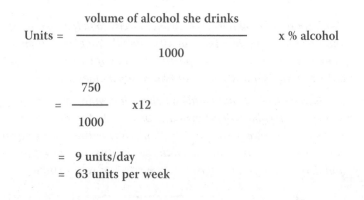

$$\text{Units} = \frac{\text{volume of alcohol she drinks}}{1000} \times \% \text{ alcohol}$$

$$= \frac{750}{1000} \times 12$$

$$= 9 \text{ units/day}$$
$$= 63 \text{ units per week}$$

Fig. 11 Volume of alcohol consumed

CLINICAL MANAGEMENT SKILLS

- She hasn't taken citalopram for 5 days. As she isn't keen on continuing the course, it is reasonable to not to prescribe any more (unless she is getting withdrawal effects).

- She would like counselling – a referral should be made. Counselling would address depression and alcohol use. Has she considered relationship counselling?

- Consider prescribing vitamin B supplements.

- Does she need time off work?

- Is she interested in self help books or websites? Would she prefer over-the-counter, rather than prescribed therapy, eg St John's Wort.

INTERPERSONAL SKILLS

- Sensitivity is crucial to gaining her trust. She must feel supported.

- How would she best like to be helped? Offer her options, eg changing antidepressants, counselling. Does she know what to expect from different treatment modalities, what they entail and how long it may take for them to work?

- Many people are embarrassed when discussing sexual matters. If she offers a cue, one approach would be to say some women have sexual problems on citalopram and ask if that applies to her.

- She should be followed up regularly.

CASE 9

INSTRUCTIONS TO CANDIDATES (CASE NOTES)

Name	Jessica Ronson
Age	26
Past medical history	Anxiety
Social history	Married, one child, 5 years old

Tip

✓ Be aware the past medical history may not bear any relationship to the presenting case.

BRAINSTORM

INSTRUCTIONS TO ROLE PLAYER (PATIENT)

NOT TO BE SEEN BY THE CANDIDATE

Opening statement:

'Hi Doctor, I need to know about meningitis.'

Patient background:

You are Jessica Ronson, you are 26 years old.

You have a history of anxiety but your symptoms are under control.

You are worried about your son, Alfie. Alfie is normally well.

One of his classmates was diagnosed with meningitis 2 weeks ago. She will be fine and the children in her class, including Alfie, were given the all clear by Public Health.

You are confused about how meningitis may present.

You heard someone say; if he doesn't have a rash it means he doesn't have meningitis, but one of the mums at school said that was wrong.

You are sure that people with meningitis also have a headache.

You have heard that the vaccination won't fully protect him against meningitis. You would like to know if that's true and why?

NOTES

DATA-GATHERING, TECHNICAL AND ASSESSMENT SKILLS

- Finding out what happened to Alfie's classmate would be a good starting point.

- Has he had his Meningitis C vaccination?

- You may want to check his medical history, is he immunocompromised, eg splenectomy?

- What does she understand about meningococcal disease?

CLINICAL MANAGEMENT SKILLS

- Much of this consultation will revolve around delivering information in a way she understands.

- The description of meningitis, septicaemia and the differences between the two conditions should be discussed.

- In particular, the misnomer that the absence of a rash excludes a diagnosis of meningitis should be explored.

- A more general discussion about what to watch out for in a sick child of any cause is relevant.

NICE have guidance on the child with a fever.

INTERPERSONAL SKILLS

- What is her level of knowledge? There is little point in telling her what she already knows.

- Consider if she has any particular questions, or would she like you to tell her about meningitis is general?

- When discussing features of meningococcal disease, you should check she understands what you mean.

- Have you relieved her fears?

Tip

✓ **Check that you understand the patient and the patient understands you**

- She shouldn't be made to feel ignorant and should be given the opportunity to ask questions.

- Offering a leaflet about the features of meningitis and meningococcal septicaemia will help reiterate what you have said.

- Suggest she can give you a call at the surgery if she has further questions.

- You may offer to arrange an evening meeting at the local school to discuss meningitis with parents and teachers.

CHAPTER 6

PHYSICAL SIGNS IN CHILDREN WITH MENINGOCOCCAL DISEASE

ORGAN SYSTEM	SEPTICAEMIA	MENINGITIS
RESPIRATORY	• Increased respiratory rate and breathing occur early, secondary to acidosis and hypoxia as circulatory failure develops	• No changes early in disease • Abnormal breathing patterns seen late with critically raised intracranial pressure. (Vary from hyperventilation to Cheyne-Stokes breathing or apnoea)
CARDIOVASCULAR	Careful examination of this system is the key to recognition of septicaemia. Clinical features of circulatory failure (shock) develops: • Tachycardia is an early and important sign • Peripheral vasoconstriction results in pallor, cold hands and feet, and mottling • Capillary refill time >2 seconds on forehead or sternum is abnormal, ≥ 4 seconds on peripheries in conjunction with other signs suggests shock • BP is normal until late in septicaemia. Hypotension is a pre-terminal sign	• No changes early in disease • Later, raised intracranial pressure leads to bradycardia and hypertension
CNS	• Children have a normal conscious level until late in the illness and they may appear alert and responsive • Hypoxia and hypoperfusion eventually lead to a decreased conscious level: this is a late and pre-terminal sign in shock • NO neck stiffness or photophobia occurs in septicaemia	CNS function most likely to be abnormal • Irritability, drowsiness, confusion and decreased conscious level as intracranial pressure rises. Babies may have a vacant expression/full fontanelle. Teenagers can become confused and combative. • Neck stiffness and photophobia are uncommon signs in early meningitis in young children. Overall, one-third of patients with meningitis lack neck stiffness.
RENAL	• Decreased urine output occurs early in shock	• No change in meningitis
DEATH	Results from cardiovascular failure (shock)	Results from raised intracranial pressure

Meningitis Research Foundation 11/2003

Normal values of vital signs from Advanced Paediatric Life Support Manual			
Age (years)	Heart Rate per minute	Respiratory Rate per minute	Systolic Blood Pressure
<1	110–160	30–40	70–90
1–2	100–150	25–35	80–95
2–5	95–140	25–30	80–100
5–12	80–120	20–25	90–110
Over 12	60–100	15–20	100–120

RASH: The rash of meningococcal disease can start as a blanching rash in up to a third of patients: remember to check for underlying signs of meningitis and septicaemia in children who present with a maculopapular rash.

Patients with meningitis tend to have a more scanty (or absent) rash than those with septicaemia. Ideally, the whole skin surface of a febrile patient without an obvious cause for fever should be checked.

Benzylpenicillin dosage (BNF)
(except in severe penicillin allergy)
Adult and child aged 10 or older: 1200 mg
Child 1–9 years: 600 mg
Infant: 300 mg

www.meningitis.org

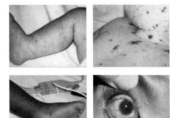

Clockwise from left: Maculopapular rash with scanty petechiae, Classic purpuric rash, Purpuric rash on dark skin, Petechial rash in conjunctivae

Fig. 12 Meningitis Research Foundation – Physical Signs in Children with Meningococcal Disease

CHAPTER 6

SIGNS TO LOOK OUT FOR IN MENINGITIS: RAPID DIAGNOSIS AND TREATMENT OF MENINGOCOCCAL DISEASE IS VITAL

Meningococcal disease is the leading infectious cause of childhood death in the UK. Around half of cases occur in children aged four years or under, although peaks are seen in teenagers and the elderly.

There are at least 13 different serotypes of *Neisseria meningitidis*, the causative agent, although most cases of meningococcal disease in the UK are caused by B or C strains. Introduction of the MenC vaccine in 1999 resulted in a marked decrease in the number of cases.

Meningococcal disease may cause septicaemia, meningitis or both. The organism may also cause arthritis, osteomyelitis or ophthalmic complications.

The early stages of meningococcal disease may present as non-specific flu-like symptoms so it is important to look for signs of septicaemia or meningitis in all febrile patients without obvious infection.

MENINGOCOCCAL SEPTICAEMIA

Meningococcal septicaemia is an emergency and is fatal in around 20 per cent of cases. A high index of suspicion and thorough examination are required when children present with signs of septicaemia.

A diagnostic tool such as the Glasgow meningococcal septicaemia prognostic score can help identify those children requiring immediate emergency treatment.

Bacterial death in the blood triggers a massive inflammatory reaction with failure of the endothelium and the clotting cascade. This produces the classic non-blanching purpuric rash of meningococcal septicaemia. In up to a third of cases the rash is maculopapular.

CHAPTER 6

Early symptoms include tachycardia, increased respiratory rate and peripheral vasoconstriction. Other features include hypoxia and oliguria. Abdominal pain, sometimes with diarrhoea, may be present and joint and bone pains can be severe.

The peripheries may be cool and mottled. A capillary refill time greater than two seconds on the sternum or forehead is abnormal while one of four seconds or more in the peripheries is suggestive of shock.

Hypotension and altered consciousness are late signs in children. Without treatment, organ failure and cardiovascular collapse will eventually lead to death in these cases.

MENINGITIS

Meningitis has a different presentation to septicaemia and a much lower mortality rate at less than 5 per cent.

Symptoms include severe headache, impaired consciousness, photophobia and neck stiffness, although in young children both neck stiffness and photophobia occur later in the illness and up to a third do not even develop neck stiffness.

Kernig's sign may be positive. Babies may also present with a tense fontanelle, vacant stare, high pitched cry, poor feeding or a change in tone.

In older children and teenagers meningitis can cause changes in behaviour such as confusion or aggression. These signs are sometimes presumed to be alcohol related.

Meningitis may also cause raised intracranial pressure, which can eventually lead to cardiorespiratory compromise and death.

Signs of this include declining consciousness; unequal, dilated or poorly responsive pupils; hypertension; and relative bradycardia.

IMMEDIATE CARE

A child presenting with meningitis or a fever and purpuric rash should be treated for meningococcal disease without delay. Blood tests to confirm the infection can be carried out after antibiotics have been administered.

Antibiotics should be given intravenously where possible. Benzylpenicillin or cefotaxime are first-line agents.

Chloramphenicol may be used if there is a definite history of allergy to these agents. Oxygen should be given.

Treatment for sepsis may also include fluid resuscitation and inotropic support, usually within a hospital setting.

A lumbar puncture should be taken when meningitis is suspected. Treatment should also be administered where the diagnosis is unclear.

A child with worrying symptoms should be transferred to a paediatric unit via a blue-light ambulance, with a receiving team on standby.

NOTIFICATION

Meningococcal disease is a notifiable disease. The consultant in communicable disease control is responsible for ensuring that anyone who has been in close contact with the patient receives prophylaxis.

Drugs used to clear carriage include rifampicin, ciprofloxacin and ceftriaxone.

Contacts should be informed that these drugs are not used to treat infection and the signs of established meningococcal disease should be discussed with them.

By Dr R Thakkar

Reproduced with kind permission from Independent Nurse[2], April 2008

CHAPTER 6

CASE 10

INSTRUCTIONS TO CANDIDATES (CASE NOTES)

You arrive at this patient's home. She requested a home visit for abdominal pain. You have a paper summary of her notes with you. Her grandson lets you into the house.

You have a doctor's bag with standard equipment and drugs (including opiates).

Name	Mary Baron
Age	72
Past medical history	MI × 3
	Rheumatoid arthritis
	Depression
Current medication	Aspirin 75 mg od
	Ramipril 10 mg od
	Simvastatin 40 mg nocte
	Atenolol 50 mg od
	Paracetamol 1g qds
	Tramadol 50 mg qds
	Prednisolone 5 mg od
	Methotrexate 10 mg weekly
	Alendronic acid 70 mg weekly
	Folic acid 5 mg weekly
	Ibuprofen 400 mg prn
	Fluoxetine 20 mg od
Social history	Lives with grandson (age 17), recently widowed

Note: this patient has a pulse of 110/min, BP 109/40, is sweaty and has a rigid abdomen.

CHAPTER 6

BRAINSTORM

INSTRUCTIONS TO ROLE PLAYER (PATIENT)

NOT TO BE SEEN BY THE CANDIDATE

Opening statement:

'Doctor, help me, I'm in pain.'

Patient background:

You are Mary Baron, you are 72 years old.

You have severe abdominal pain.

It started suddenly about 3 hours ago.

It is above your belly button.

You have been vomiting.

You can't move because you're in too much pain.

You don't have any chest pain.

This is the worst pain you have ever experienced.

You don't have any drug allergies.

You are scared to go into hospital; you don't want to get MRSA. You agree to go when the doctor recommends it.

You are sweaty and your heart is pounding fast in your chest.

Whenever the doctor examines your stomach, it is exquisitely painful and it feels rock hard.

You can't stand the pain any more.

You think you may be having a heart attack.

NOTES

DATA-GATHERING, TECHNICAL AND ASSESSMENT SKILLS

- It is likely that this patient has a perforated peptic ulcer. She takes a number of drugs that put her at risk for peptic ulcer disease.

- As she is unwell, it is reasonable to take a quick and directed history.

- Her vital signs should be measured: temperature, pulse and blood pressure.

- Examination of her abdomen would reveal a rigid abdomen with guarding.

- Ask about chest pain, particularly given her history of coronary artery disease.

CLINICAL MANAGEMENT SKILLS

- It is clear this patient needs a surgical opinion.

- It would be appropriate to call 999.

- If she is not allergic to any medication, intramuscular/intravenous opiates and anti-emetics should be given.

Tip

   ✓ **You should not administer any drugs during the CSA.**

- The surgical team at the local hospital should be notified you are sending the patient in.

- You will have to write a letter of referral to the surgical team.

- You should wait for the ambulance to arrive; she is at risk of cardiac arrest (you would have to express that you would wait for the ambulance to the examiner).

CHAPTER 6

INTERPERSONAL SKILLS

- Both the patient and her grandson will be worried and concerned.

- Is she happy for her grandson to be present while you are talking to her?

- You will need to gain her confidence, keep cool and demonstrate you are in control.

- Even though she requires hospital management, it is important to keep her informed as to what you think is going on and why you think she requires hospital treatment.

- It would be reasonable if you ask if she has any concerns with your plan to arrange hospital management. Her concerns should be addressed and expectations discussed. This may relieve her anxiety. In addition to contracting MRSA and having a 'heart attack' she may be concerned about dying, never coming out of hospital and what may happen to her in hospital.

CASE 11

INSTRUCTIONS TO CANDIDATES (CASE NOTES)

Name	Hilary Gilligan
Age	69
Past medical history	Shingles × 2
Current medication	Nil
Social history	Married, five children

Previous consultation (one week ago):

Shingles, has had two previous episodes this year.

Right T10, for aciclovir.

Review if concerned.

BRAINSTORM

INSTRUCTIONS TO ROLE PLAYER (PATIENT)

NOT TO BE SEEN BY THE CANDIDATE

Opening statement:

'Hi Doctor, I need your advice.'

Patient background:

You are Hilary Gilligan, 69 years old.

You have shingles, diagnosed last week by another doctor at your practice.

You are worried because your daughter is pregnant and you think you may give her shingles if you see her.

She is 7 weeks pregnant.

She had chicken pox when she was a child.

You think that shingles is caught from other people with shingles.

You know there is a link between chicken pox and shingles, but you don't fully understand it.

You would like to know more about shingles.

This is your third episode of shingles this year.

You have had some weight loss and night sweats lately.

You are not stressed and can't wait to see your first grandchild.

You have been more tired lately.

Your bowel habit hasn't changed although you have had some abdominal pain.

You haven't had any bone pain.

NOTES

DATA-GATHERING, TECHNICAL AND ASSESSMENT SKILLS

- This consultation has two issues. The first focuses on the behaviour of the herpes zoster virus. The second is about the management of a patient with potential immune paresis.

- Regarding her recurrent shingles, you should consider immune paresis. Given her age group, conditions such as CLL, lymphoma, myeloma, myelodysplasia, marrow infiltration, and diabetes should be considered.

- Red flag symptoms should be sought.

- Examination of her abdomen to check for hepatosplenomegaly and lymphadenopathy shows forward and lateral thinking.

Tip

✓ Explain why you are asking questions and what you are examining for. Signposting to the patient would help them understand your thought process. For example, she may find it odd if, out of the blue, you expressed the wish to examine her abdomen when she was concerned about her daughter getting shingles. If you discussed that some patients with recurrent shingles have an enlarged spleen and you were just checking hers, she would think you are a thoughtful doctor.

CLINICAL MANAGEMENT SKILLS

- Check FBC (film for smear cells and CLL), ESR, myeloma screen, glucose. Chest X-ray (CXR) for mediatstinal lymph nodes. You are looking for conditions pre-disposing her to recurrent shingles.

INTERPERSONAL SKILLS

- It is helpful to know what the patient's current level of understanding about chicken pox and shingles is. Once this is clear, you can offer an explanation clarifying any deficiencies in her knowledge base, which is:

  - Chicken pox occurs in patients who have never been exposed to the herpes zoster virus (by exposure to chicken pox or shingles). It is unusual to get chicken pox more than once.

  - Once a patient has had chicken pox, the virus sits dormant in the spinal cord (dorsal root ganglion).

  - For many reasons, the virus can reactivate and migrate along a (sensory) nerve to cause shingles in the distribution of that nerve (dermatomal).

  - A patient with shingles can shed the (herpes zoster) virus and cause chicken pox in someone who has never had chicken pox before.

  - Pregnant women who have never had chicken pox before are at risk.

- She should not be made to feel silly.

- Checking her understanding by summarising what you have said is important.

- What are her ideas on patients who have recurrent shingles? Does she know that there may be underlying causes?

- A leaflet on shingles and chicken pox, perhaps from www.patient.co.uk would back up what you have said.

- She should be followed up to discuss her blood tests.

CHAPTER 6

CASE 12

INSTRUCTIONS TO CANDIDATES (CASE NOTES)

Name	Mary Smith
Age	63
Past medical history	OA
	Hypothyroidism
	Obesity
	Hypertension
Current medication	Paracetamol 1 g qds
	Amlodipine 5 mg od
	Levothyroxine 150 mcg od
Social history	Married, three children

Last consultation (one week ago):

Nocturia, polydypsia and weight loss. BP persistently raised > 150/90.

Plan – Check fasting blood sugar, TSH and BP with nurse, then review next week

Results:

Glucose	16.7 mmol/l
TSH	Euthyroid
BP	122/73

BRAINSTORM

INSTRUCTIONS TO ROLE PLAYER (PATIENT)

NOT TO BE SEEN BY THE CANDIDATE

Opening statement:

'I've come to get my results Doctor!'

Patient background:

You are Mary Smith, you are 63 years old.

You live with your husband, who is disabled after his stroke last year, and your youngest son who has recently finished his university degree.

You have been losing weight recently *which you were pleased about.* However, you also noticed you were drinking more than normal and passing a lot of urine.

You are concerned that your levothyroxine dose isn't right.

You have osteoarthritis.

You have had hypothyroidism for 15 years. *It runs in the family, both you mother and your sister have it.*

You have been more tired recently, which you don't quite understand. Last time, when your levothyroxine dose was too high, you didn't suffer fatigue.

Your bowel habit is normal and you're not sensitive to extremes of temperature.

You try to eat healthily to help control your blood pressure which has been hard to control.

You don't smoke.

Once you were given the diagnosis of diabetes you become concerned about having to check your blood sugars every day and having to inject yourself with insulin. You don't know exactly what diabetes is or what the complications are.

NOTES

DATA-GATHERING, TECHNICAL AND ASSESSMENT SKILLS

- This patient has type 2 diabetes. She is symptomatic with a raised fasting blood sugar above 7.0 mmol/l. Had she been asymptomatic, she would require a further confirmatory test.

- Much of the consultation will revolve around educating the patient.

- It would be helpful to confirm the history and to consider what her concerns are. You can then break the bad news bearing in mind her health beliefs. Many patients are fearful of being diabetic.

- Features of diabetes itself should be asked for, polyuria, polydypsia, weight loss, and fatigue.

- She should be asked about any symptoms of cardiovascular, eye and neuropathic disease.

- You should discuss lifestyle; does she smoke, what is her diet like, does she exercise?

- It is important to check her blood pressure.

CLINICAL MANAGEMENT SKILLS

- Holistic and systematic care of diabetic patients is essential. Most practices will have a diabetes clinic and may have a doctor and/or a nurse who takes a special interest in the subject. NICE published guidance on management of type 2 diabetes in May 2008. They highlight the importance of patient education and lifestyle advice.

- Are there any diabetes patient groups locally and would she like to attend?

- She should be put on the diabetes register and be recalled for regular review.

DERBY VOCATIONAL TRAINING SCHEME FOR GENERAL PRACTICE

CHAPTER 6

- Lifestyle is a major part of diabetes management. It is important to impress on her the importance of losing weight and how this may benefit her arthritis as well as her diabetes.

- Further bloods are required: HbA1c, u/e and fasting lipids, with appropriate follow-up for further management.

- The nurse should weigh her and repeat her blood pressure when she takes her blood.

- Urinary albumin:creatinine ratio (ACR) is required. She should be asked to drop a first-pass (rather than mid-stream) urine sample into the practice. Does she know why you are checking her urine?

- She may be commenced on a statin as evidence suggests diabetic patients are at as much risk of ischaemic cardiac events as patients who have an established diagnosis of coronary artery disease.

- Blood pressure should be appropriately controlled in diabetes.

Tip

✓ **Use the BNF or MIMS (if available) during the consultation as you would in a routine surgery. They often give useful clinical pointers and guidelines if you're stuck!**

- She should be referred to the retinopathy clinic for regular assessment. Explain why this is important and check out whether she is happy for you to go ahead with the referral.

INTERPERSONAL SKILLS

- Explaining a new diagnosis of diabetes brings with it a raft of issues, many of which have been discussed earlier. You won't be able to discuss all of the issues in a 10 minute consultation. It is far better to concentrate on a few major points, so she feels satisfied and empowered, than to deliver a unilateral speech on diabetes leaving her feeling overwhelmed.

CHAPTER 6

- What does she think diabetes is? Does she know why people get it? Does she understand why it is important to treat it properly?

- For many people, diabetes is a mystery while others are well aware of its complications. It is important to assess what her level of knowledge is and to pitch your consultation accordingly. She should be educated as much as possible.

- What are her concerns? Insulin dependence is a common concern.

- She may become upset and sensitivity should be demonstrated.

- It is important to get her on board with treatment in order to optimise her care.

- Can you offer any leaflets or websites if she has access to the internet?

- Follow-up is important, she is likely to have many more questions once she leaves your consulting room and you will need to discuss the results of the investigations you have arranged. You may want to offer a double (20 minute) appointment next time and ask her to write down any questions she may have.

NICE, TYPE 2 DIABETES, MAY 2008

KEY POINTS:

- Self monitoring and education important

- Patient-centred care

- Dietary and lifestyle advice

  - eg smoking, exercise

  - advise low GI foods, oily fish, reduce dairy products

- When initiating insulin the following are important: education, telephone support, self-monitoring and management of hypoglycaemic episodes

- Be sensitive to patients' cultural, linguistic, cognitive needs
- HbA1c general target 6.5% or less
- Target may be higher based on discussion with individual
- Monitor HbA_{1c} 2–6 monthly if sugars unstable or 6 monthly if stable
- Self monitoring for all patients, if they are able, unless they are just controlled on diet or metformin
- Advise self monitoring of glucose to assess safety, eg when driving
- Patients should have an overall management plan.

BLOOD GLUCOSE LOWERING THERAPY

- If HbA1c > 6.5% despite lifestyle intervention – start metformin
- If HbA1c remains > 6.5% or if metformin not tolerated – add in/start sulfonylurea
- If HbA1c > 7.5% – add in glitazone (pioglitazone) or insulin

METFORMIN:

- Increase dose over a few weeks – minimises GI side effects
- Care if creatinine > 130 µmol/L or eGFR < 45 ml/min
- Stop if creatinine > 150 µmol/L or eGFR < 30 ml/min
- BMJ, 2007 – metformin does not, on its own, cause lactic acidosis.

SULFONYLUREA:

- Warn about hypoglycaemia.

GLITAZONES:

- Diabetes Care, 2007 – increased risk of heart failure.

BLOOD PRESSURE MANAGEMENT:

- If end organ damage, aim BP < 130/80 mmHg, otherwise < 140/80 mmHg. The British Hypertension Society recommends < 130/80 mmHg generally for diabetes

- If not hypertensive and no renal disease, review annually

- If BP > 150/90 mmHg repeat in 1 month

- If BP > 130/80 (if end organ damage) or > 140/80 mmHg, repeat in 2 months

- Use ACE-I/CCB as appropriate.

LIPID MANAGEMENT:

- Assess CVD risk annually including lipid profile

- Simvastatin first line, to 40 mg.

ANTITHROMBOTIC THERAPY:

- If over 50 yrs and BP < 145/90 mmHg

- If < 50 yrs and other significant CVD risk factors.

RENAL DISEASE:

- Annual ACR – first pass sample

- Annual creatinine and eGFR estimation

- Microalbuminuria if at least one ACR test is abnormal (> 2.5 mg/mmol for men or > 3.5 mg/mmol for women)

- Consider non-diabetic causes of renal disease

- Treat nephropathy with ACE-I and aim for BP < 130/80 mmHg.

CHAPTER 6

CASE 13

INSTRUCTIONS TO CANDIDATES (CASE NOTES)

You have never met this patient before.

Name   Brian Dover

Age   48

Social history   Works as a carpenter, never smoked

Last entry in notes (2 weeks ago):

Home visit: Acute shortness of breath

                      Looks unwell

                      Respiratory rate 40/min

                      Pulse 120/min

                      Creps bibasally

                      Impression – acute LVF

                      Plan – refer to medics

Handwritten discharge letter from hospital:

Acute LVF, secondary to viral infection

Angio: NAD, echo: moderate left ventricular systolic dysfunction

Medications on discharge: Ramipril 5 mg od, GP, please check u/e

                            Bisoprolol 5 mg od

                            Furosemide 20 mg od

Review, 2 months in clinic with repeat echo. Cardiac rehab.

BRAINSTORM

INSTRUCTIONS TO ROLE PLAYER (PATIENT)

NOT TO BE SEEN BY THE CANDIDATE

Opening statement:

'Hi Doctor! I've come to get my pills!'

Patient background:

You are Brian Dover, you are 48 years old.

You became suddenly short of breath 2 weeks ago and called for an urgent home visit.

You saw your usual GP, Dr Thakkar, he sent you into hospital.

You went to hospital for 5 days. You initially spent hours in Accident and Emergency and were then admitted to the cardiac ward.

You had blood tests, X-rays and a specialist doctor scanned your heart. You also had a test, 'angio' something, to see if you have blocked arteries in your heart. Luckily that was normal.

The cardiologist said Dr Thakkar was spot on; that you had LVF and it was it was probably due to a virus.

You have no idea what LVF means.

The hospital doctors gave you lots of medicines into your veins to help your breathing. You were given tablets to take when you are at home.

You don't drink alcohol or smoke.

You were given 2 weeks supply of your pills and you have come to get some more.

You don't know how long you have to take the medicines for.

You can't remember the drug doses, but you follow the instructions on the box.

You have had today's drugs, but don't have any left for tomorrow. You forgot to bring the boxes with you.

You are not quite sure what the drugs do.

CHAPTER 6

> *You haven't felt breathless at all since you left hospital.*
>
> *You don't get breathless when you lie flat in bed or when you walk to the local shops.*
>
> *You are worried what the future holds.*
>
> *The hospital will be starting an exercise programme for you soon.*

NOTES

DATA-GATHERING, TECHNICAL AND ASSESSMENT SKILLS

- The hospital discharge summary (see case notes) provides key information about his diagnosis, medication and follow-up.

- The main focus of this case is to ensure he understands his condition and its management (all this information is provided on the discharge summary).

- Does he know what happened to him?

- How is his breathing now?

- Does he have any symptoms of breathlessness – on exertion, at rest, orthopnoea, paroxysmal nocturnal dynpnoea?

- Is he getting side effects of drugs? (Look in the BNF if you can't remember although this may take up valuable time).

- Check his pulse, blood pressure, auscultate his heart sounds and lung fields and check for pitting oedema.

CHAPTER 6

- Ask about what drugs he is on and if he knows what they are for.

- Does he know the drug doses and when to take them?

- Is he aware of how to get more drugs (repeat prescription system)?

- Does he know what the follow-up plans are – cardiac exercise programme and clinic follow-up?

CLINICAL MANAGEMENT SKILLS

- Inform him of what happened and why.

- Explain why he has been prescribed his drugs, what side effects to watch out for and how he can get more.

- Organise U/E and explain why this is important. Explain you will contact him if you are concerned about the results.

- Explain what he should do if he gets breathless.

- Prescribe the drugs he requires.

INTERPERSONAL SKILLS

- Getting the story from the patient, about what happened in hospital may provide you with information about his understanding, health beliefs, and concerns. Many people are fearful of heart disease.

- He has been through a frightening experience. To acknowledge how frightening this must have been for him may offer a channel for him to express his concerns.

- What are his ideas as to what happened? Did he think he had a heart attack? Does he know what LVF means? What is his view when you use the word 'failure'?

- What are his expectations? Does he expect to achieve a full recovery?

- It would be difficult to offer an accurate prognosis, particularly without a formal hospital letter with the test results. It is reasonable to be honest and say you don't have enough information at this stage; the hospital team will be able to provide more information on how he is doing once the second scan has been done in a few weeks time.

- Offer hope rather than doom and gloom.

- Suggest he comes back in a few weeks, perhaps after he is seen in clinic, to see how he is doing may offer added support.

- Agree a plan of action between you and the patient that suits you both, eg follow-up, prescribing of drugs.

- It is important to summarise what you have said and check his understanding.

- Give him the opportunity to ask further questions which may be discussed at a later date, he may think of questions once he leaves the consulting room.

REFERENCES

(1) *Consent: patients and doctors making decisions together* reviewed by Dr Raj Thakkar, GMC Today, May/June 2008 p6.

(2) Thakkar R (2008) Signs to look out for in meningitis, Rapid diagnosis and treatment of meningococcal disease is vital. Independent Nurse, 7–10 April 2008 p22.

Chapter 7
What next?

The nMRCGP® assesses the ability of a candidate to practise safely and effectively as an independent GP. The CSA aims to reflect everyday general practice cases rather than esoteric medicine, and preparation should be an ongoing process that occurs throughout GP training rather than a cramming exercise two weeks before the examination.

Between now and the examination try to treat every patient you see as a CSA case. Consult in a patient-centred way using recognised consultation models (eg Pendelton *et al.*, Neighbour, Silverman). Read up on the knowledge (eg guidelines) required to manage the problems you come across during your consultations. Reflect on how you managed each case; how could you do better next time? What are your learning needs and how can you address these deficiencies?

The CSA is more than a test of consultation skills and disease management, it also tests examination skills. Unlike the MRCP, the clinical examinations required within the CSA are likely to focus on symptoms rather than systems. This being the case, in addition to considering the questions you may need to ask, it is useful to practice examination of a patient with specific symptoms such as headaches, breathlessness, tiredness, and so on. You will also have to demonstrate you can use medical equipment proficiently, such as peak flow meters, inhalers, and obstetric calendars.

How can you know if you are consulting to the right standard? Make use of the consultation observational tool (COT). Organise joint surgeries with your trainer and the other GPs in your practice. This will demonstrate different techniques and consulting styles that you can adopt. Your trainer can also give you feedback and discuss ways in which you can improve your skills. Videoing your consultations and watching them back on your own, with peers or with your trainer is a powerful tool. It will help you identify your strengths and more importantly, your weaknesses. You can also review the video consultations offered as free 'Online Extras' in conjunction with this book – see www.pastest.co.uk/online extras.

Role playing cases with a colleague playing the patient and another observing is invaluable and provides practice under 'examination conditions.'

The nMRCGP should be a joy to prepare for. A planned approach, consistent application and dedication are required for success. Reflect on your learning needs, make use of the teachers around you and regularly visit the RCGP website.

Whichever way you approach the nMRCGP, remember your registrar year is supposed to be exciting, enlightening and above all, enjoyable! Good luck!

CHAPTER 7

INDEX